Karen Blackford
838-6026

W9-BSE-357

CHILD-BIRTH AT HOME

CHILD-BIRTH AT HOME

by Marion Sousa

PRENTICE-HALL, INC.
Englewood Cliffs, N.J.

Childbirth at Home
by Marion Sousa

Printed in the United States of America
Prentice-Hall International, Inc., London
Prentice-Hall of Australia, Pty. Ltd., Sydney
Prentice-Hall of Canada, Ltd., Toronto
Prentice-Hall of India Private Ltd., New Delhi
Prentice-Hall of Japan, Inc., Tokyo

10 9 8 7 6 5 4 3 2 1

Library of Congress Cataloging in Publication Data

Sousa, Marion,
    Childbirth at home.

    Bibliography: p.
    Includes Index.
    1. Natural childbirth. I. Title.
DNLM: 1. Natural childbirth. WQ150 S725c
RG661.S68   618.4'5   75-17805
ISBN 0-13-130369-4

FOREWORD

The young, child-bearing people of today are staging a revolution against the outmoded, tired, old, conventional form of "knock-'em-out, drag-'em-out" hospital obstetrics of yesterday. Marion Sousa is a pioneer leader and capable spokesman for her group and she has gone to considerable trouble to delve into available literature and medical research to back up her convictions with scientific facts and adequate references. I found her book refreshing in its thoroughness.

Those followers of true, natural, unmedicated childbirth who are aware of my writings and teachings as president of the American Academy of Husband-Coached Childbirth may be astounded that I was asked to write the foreword to a book advocating childbirth at home as I have long been "agin it." But Mrs. Sousa noted that I had asked Dr. Ashley Montagu, who has long been for home births, to write the foreword to my book *Husband-Coached Childbirth,* so she decided to utilize the same pattern. I am proud to cooperate; her book is an excellent one and the best yet on home births.

Actually, I cannot escape involvement. The form of un-medicated, true, natural childbirth based upon the instinctual

behavior of fellow mammals that our academy teaches is the
ideal conduct for bearing a child at home as it has proven to
have the shortest labors, the least complications, and the most
capable management of these complications when they do
occur.

Not only do most home births utilize the "Bradley
Method," but I blushingly admit that several of our certified
childbirth educators, against our advice, have served as lay
mid-wives at home births in areas where hospitals and doctors are rigidly adhering to the old routine of drugs and
anesthesia for all cases.

One can very much admire Mrs. Sousa's courage and
determination to buck the system she sincerely feels is pitifully
wrong, inadequate, and, as she adroitly proves in this book,
definitely harmful to babies and parents. I am in complete
agreement with every point she makes that most hospitals are
great, gaunt, marble mausoleums where obstetrics is looked
upon as a disease of nine months duration.

Then why am I "agin it"? Because I feel it is an admission
of failure in our determination to change and humanize hospitals. Young parents must not cower before the domineer-
ing, bluffing, big, pompous medical "sheriffs" whose
"You're in a heap-of-trouble, son!" I know can be overcome
by organized efforts of determined consumers. You *can* fight
medical "city halls" and make maternity hospitals homelike.
Difficult as it seems, superficially, it has been done in some
areas already. Our childbirth educators carry consumer
power wherein any area hospital that makes its maternity
ward homelike, that includes husbands at all times, that encourages unmedicated births with immediate breast feeding,
etc., will be "girl-cotted" by many referrals of patients. Any
hospital that rigidly adheres to outmoded obstetrics will be
boycotted into bankruptcy. Hospitals and doctors are public
servants and should serve consumer wants; if they don't, they
can be changed.

Pregnant couples fly into Denver to utilize our changed
and humanized hospital, have their babies unmedicated by

true natural childbirth, breast-feed them on the delivery
table, walk back to the recovery room after drinking their
orange juice, and go home in two hours. They thereby reap
the many benefits Mrs. Sousa's fine book itemizes with the
added safety of being where the doctor has all his tools of
trade to manage immediately any unforeseen and unexpected complications.

I do not encourage coming to Denver to do this but
verbally "spank" them and tell them to go back home and
change their own hospitals. The directors and founders of
our Academy in California, Marjie & Jay Hathaway, were one
such couple who heeded the spanking and did just that. They
changed many local hospitals through organized public ap-
peals. Indeed, part of our training of Bradley Method teach-
ers includes the Hathaways' teaching on how to change hospitals in your area.

Mrs. Sousa's book serves the noble purpose of bringing
problem hospitals before the public eye. From this public
awareness, steps will be taken to initiate change.

As a former farmer, if I had separated animal babies
from their mothers as soon as they were born, put the babies
in a box with a glass window and let the mother only look
through the window at them for two or three days, I would
have been arrested for cruelty to animals. Yet this is what
hospital "routines" do to humans. I know of no reason why
pediatricians cannot walk from room to room when making
rounds, as obstetricians do, to see their patients and leave
human babies in their mothers' arms where they belong instead of putting the babies in a big box called the new-born
nursery, or more appropriately the "kid concentration camp."

Difficult as changing and humanizing hospitals appears
to be, it is still easier to make a hospital homelike than to make
a home hospital-like. We can then keep separate the role of
the doctor from that of the lover, the husband. The doctor is a
lousy lover, and the lover, if complications should arise, would
be a lousy doctor, in my opinion. Each is needed in his respec-
tive role as Mrs. Sousa's book so well illustrates.

If a pregnant couple (parents do come in pairs) are living in an area where hospitals have not changed, and in the short time before birth is expected the hospital is unlikely to change, and a humanized hospital is not within driving distance, then Mrs. Sousa's book serves as a thorough guide to home birth. Study it carefully as her points are well-taken.

Robert A. Bradley, M.D., President
American Academy of Husband-
Coached Childbirth

ACKNOWLEDGMENTS

Many people helped me see this book through from its conception to its eventual birth! Thanks go to my husband, who not only delivered our last two children, but also did plenty of baby-sitting and dishwashing so I could get the book written. I'm tremendously grateful to all the other mothers, fathers, midwives and doctors who cared enough about home births to share their experiences with me. I also appreciate the professional criticism supplied by several lawyers, a few nurses, and a theologian.

The staff at the North Highlands, California, County Library was extremely responsive to my multitudinous requests for hard-to-get reference material. During the two years I worked on the book, a number of writers and writing students in Sacramento, California, were kind enough to supply me with innumerable articles and free criticism; both were very helpful!

North Highlands. California

ix

INTRODUCTION

"Have a baby at home? Isn't that what some of those hippies do in California?"

They certainly do, but so do an increasing number of women from upper- and middle-class America. I'm one of them. As the wife of an Air Force officer and the mother of five young children, I hardly qualify for membership in the counterculture. Yet we had our last two babies at home—by choice, not by chance. Furthermore, only my husband was present when the babies were born. Childbirth, we thought, should be a family affair.

Emotionally, we found that having a baby at home proved superior to hospital delivery in countless ways. And after starting research for this book, I discovered that home birth might well be superior physically, too. I pursued childbirth information through the fields of sociology, anthropology, psychology, and biology. Evidence from all these disciplines strongly suggested that our national custom of confining normal births to the hospital is definitely unhealthy and possibly dangerous.

The first three chapters of this book, therefore, reveal the deleterious results of hospital delivery. Like a stone which causes ripples when cast into a pond, our conventional maternity care system produces unhappy consequences first in the mother and her baby, then in her husband and her other children, and finally in society itself. As anthropologist Lester D. Hazell explains in *Commonsense Childbirth,* "for some of us our present American way of birth is totally destructive. . . . On all of us, men, women and children, it inflicts scars."

An American woman who is pregnant now, however, may feel that she simply has no other choice but to deliver in a hospital. Does she actually have no alternative? This question is explored in Chapter 4. The following chapters confront equally controversial issues. Who should, and who should *not* consider having babies at home? And who ought to attend the birth? Surprisingly enough, the man who is always considered the ultimate authority in pregnancy and childbirth manuals may not be the best choice of attendant for a home birth.

Doctors should have no quarrel with this book, though. There are many women who clearly need medical attention during childbirth. Since the average obstetrician spends about eight years learning how to take care of the 5 percent or so of mothers who present complications, he is obviously the person who should provide this care. Furthermore, an advantageous effect of increased home deliveries would be the freeing of the obstetrician from these routine births. He would be able to devote his full attention to the patients who truly need his specialized skills. Could such a change possibly be one of the steps we should take in order to improve our appalling infant mortality rate?

This book, however, is primarily for the large majority of women whose babies are born normally. More of these women ought to realize that there is no law saying they must have their babies in the hospital. In fact, if more American mothers-to-be were completely aware of the hidden hazards of the average maternity ward, they might be a lot more hesitant about meekly handing their bodies over to the hospital's care. An expectant mother should go to the hospital to have her baby not because of social pressure, but because she really needs (or wants) the kind of attention the hospital offers.

Parents who feel that the birth of their child ought to be a family event, rather than a surgical operation, can find enough facts and guidelines in this book to help them make an informed decision about where to have their baby. My husband and I decided that the privacy of our bedroom would provide the most natural setting for a natural birth. Whoever feels the same way can read the final chapters. They explain how to prepare for what has been described as the "zenith of the creative experience"—childbirth.

CONTENTS

CHILD-
BIRTH
AT
HOME

1

WHY HOME CHILDBIRTH?

If you are about to have a baby, you are one of the vast majority of American women who will go to a hospital for its birth. Naturally, you want the best care for your baby and yourself. But you probably do not realize that when you sign into the hospital, you will be entering an atmosphere that is "almost criminally neglectful of the most fundamental needs of both."

Although I heartily agree with these words, I didn't say them first. They were written in 1969 by Dr. John S. Miller, chief of the obstetrics and gynecology service of French Hospital in San Francisco, California. At the same time, Dr. Miller revealed that he was receiving at least three requests per week for home deliveries. These requests, in Dr. Miller's opinion, come from "very knowledgeable people who know the modern obstetrical scene and choose to say 'No, thanks.' "

This book is being written for those people. It's aimed especially at all women who want to run their own deliveries instead of being "treated like dumb animals and subjected to unnecessary suffering and embarrassment."[1] The following chapters offer a concrete alternative to anyone who agrees that childbirth ought to be a warm, family-centered experience—not an impersonal operation carried out in an assembly-line atmosphere.

American women are finally beginning to express their rage over the way they have been denied control of their own labors and deliveries. In 1971, the Boston Women's Health Book Collective articulated this anger in *Our Bodies, Ourselves.* The Boston group's bitter description of hospital childbirth procedures awoke unhappy memories in thousands of American mothers. This is what the authors wrote about today's childbirth customs in the hospital.

> There we are separated at a crucial time from family and friends. We and our present children suffer from this sudden absence. In the hospital we are depersonalized; usually our clothes and personal effects, right down to glasses and hairpins, are taken away. We lose our identity. We are expected to be passive and acquiescent and to make no trouble. (Passivity is considered a sign of maturity.) We are expected to depend not on ourselves but on doctors. Most often for the doctor's convenience, we are given drugs to "ease" our labor. . . . After our baby is born s/he is taken away for an hour, for a day, or longer. We pay a lot of money for our hospital space, sometimes more than we can afford.

In 1975, the fee for the average maternity stay at a California hospital was around $500. This includes mother and baby care for a normal, uncomplicated birth. It does not, however, include the doctor's bill. Naturally, the obstetrical fee can vary from about $200 to over $2,000—depending upon where the doctor practices. The going rate in New York City, for example, seems to range from $500 to $750 for a normal delivery. Therefore, an average American mother who does not carry medical maternity insurance must pay around $1,000 to have her baby in the hospital. (For many metropolitan areas the total is closer to $2,000.) Somehow, this seems like quite a lot to pay for a routine birth

—something which nature has been doing free for other, less technically advanced peoples.

Some women mistakenly assume their medical health insurance will cover their maternity costs. Unfortunately, many health plans now pick up only a small portion of these bills. Blue Cross, for example, may pay as little as $150. And most health insurance plans only provide maternity benefits if the mother was enrolled at the time of her baby's conception. Since statistics say that up to 50% of first babies are now conceived before their parents get married, many of these births are excluded from health insurance benefits—even if the parents subsequently join a medical care plan.

During the past several years, however, consumerism has been raising its logical head. American wives have begun to both vocalize their disgust and to seek a constructive alternative. When a Port Angeles, Washington, housewife delivered her fifth baby at home, she explained why in no uncertain terms.

"The cost of a hospital is so high that you can't afford to go unless you are rich or on welfare," she complained. "The charge now is $27.50 per day to take care of the baby. I think this is a little high for changing diapers!"

As recently as 1968, maternity care—(including the obstetrician's fee)—could be purchased for under $500.[2] The same care now averages more than $1,000, even though the length of the average maternity stay has been *shortened* from five to three days. At this rate, the typical maternity fee will probably exceed $1,500 long before 1980.

Do these skyrocketing prices reflect a rising level of quality in American obstetrical care? Even knowledgeable obstetricians do not say so; our newborn mortality rate has risen substantially since 1950.[3] By 1972, the United States had dropped from sixth to fifteenth place; that is, fourteen other countries save more newborns' lives than we do. Most of the countries that outdo us, such as England, Holland, Norway and Sweden, enjoy a level of medical and technological development which equals ours. None of them, however, delegates maternity care completely to its medical community as we do. Could their systems of home delivery be why they do so much better at saving infants' lives? Holland, for example, usually places first or second when the annual infant mortality rates are published. Yet *more than seven out of ten Dutch babies are born at home.*[4]

In our own country, what hope do we have of improving our shameful infant mortality rate? Very little, in the opinion of one noted obstetrician who was also Special Assistant to the President on Population Problems. According to Dr. Louis Hellman, by 1980 about 40 percent of American babies will be born on "wards of municipal and community hospitals in which there are not and will not be enough physicians to deliver the babies or even enough to provide adequate supervision."[5]

When it comes to childbirth, most Americans still equate going to the hospital to receiving the best care. Yet one out of three of our hospitals does not meet the minimum standards set by the Joint Committee on Accreditation of Hospitals. If a woman has a baby in a small hospital which does not do many deliveries, she will not receive the best maternity care. For a normal birth, the lower quality of care will not make that much difference. If the birth is complicated, however, it can make all the difference in the world.

In 1967 the American College of Obstetricians and Gynecologists (ACOG) found that many hospitals which lack accreditation required over forty minutes to prepare for an emergency Caesarean section. But a good hospital, such as the Yale-New Haven Medical Center, is always prepared for a Caesarean, so the operation itself can be performed in less than five minutes. Furthermore, almost half of the smaller hospitals couldn't give a blood transfusion with less than thirty minutes' notice.[6] Yet the health of mothers and babies may depend on the speed and efficiency with which such lifesaving procedures are performed.

Let's take a look at the man who worries most about obstetrical care. Besides scraping up enough money to pay for his wife's hospital stay, how does the average husband share in the birth of his child? If his wife receives the conventional style of maternity care, he will participate by watching television in a waiting room. Separation of husband and wife has been the rule in American obstetrics, despite the warning of a minority group of perceptive doctors that the "husband's role, as partner in parenthood, is to provide his wife with the comfort and strength of his presence."[7]

Donna and Rodger Ewy, authors of *Preparation for Childbirth,* tell husbands that by being directly committed to share in the birth, they will gain increased respect and love from their wives. A five-year study by psychologist Deborah Tanzer came to the same conclusion. After comparing "natural childbirth" mothers with mothers who had their babies by conventional methods, Dr. Tanzer found that when the husbands took an active part in labor and delivery, their wives described them as "strong, positive, competent, sharing, and supporting." Husbands who were not present during childbirth, though, were described by their wives as "largely weak, impotent, and childlike."

The surveys taken by Tanzer presented many other significant discoveries about the importance of the husband's presence during birth. The women who experienced natural childbirth with their husbands present, for example, tended to feel extremely happy and triumphant afterwards. The vast majority of mothers who had their babies conventionally, on the other hand, felt confused, lethargic, disoriented, and even somewhat anxious when they awoke. One of Tanzer's most interesting findings connected the childbirth experience with psychological growth. The women who described their deliveries as emotionally positive, or "peak experiences," were the women whose husbands had been with them for the birth.

"The husband's presence would seem a crucial factor in making childbirth a psychologically positive time, as seen by the fact that the women's perceptions of the world were far 'healthier' when husbands were present," concluded Dr. Tanzer.[8]

Emphasizing the importance of the husband's support during the entire birth process, the president of the International Childbirth Education Association points out that "it is at this time that the whole framework is laid down for his relationship to his wife as the father of their children." Psychiatrist Joost Meerlo explains why mental health professionals feel the same.

> The psychological impact of the father on the emotional development of the child has long been overlooked . . . The example set by the father is vital for shaping the destiny and eventual emotional independence of the adult to be.
>
> This joint relationship of parents with the child begins at birth. As a matter of fact, if the husband is absent at the supreme moment when a woman gives birth, it may have an adverse effect on her. Later on it may not be easy for the husband to reclaim his place, now usurped during his wife's labor by substitute figures (the obstetrician, the family doctor, the anesthetist.)[9]

In spite of all this evidence, and in the face of a growing demand for both parents to participate in the birth of their child, most American hospitals find it too inconvenient to provide a meaningful role for the husband. With their weak excuses about hospital regulations and policy, some obstetricians sound almost like certain garage service managers who just can't allow the customer to see his own car being worked on. "Company policy" or some vague insurance regulation can always be cited as the reason. When this happens, the consumer clearly has a right to be suspicious. He would be naïve not to suspect that either the work is being done in a slipshod way, or that he's being grossly overcharged for the simple tasks that actually are done.

Just as Americans have become more consumer-conscious in the marketplace, they have become more knowledgeable about the quality of the medical care they pay for. When an obstetrician gives a vague alibi about the husband's violating the sterile delivery room, today's man may retort that having a baby is hardly a surgical operation. Or he may point out that in well over 60,000 deliveries when husbands were present, there was no increase of infections.

"If they won't let me be there, maybe it's because they don't want me to see the things they're going to do to my wife," figures one husband. ". . . and if that's the case, I'd be crazy to let her go there at all."

At least one reputable obstetrician admits that this line of reasoning may be valid. In *Husband-Coached Childbirth,* Dr. Robert A. Bradley remarks that he wouldn't even allow a stray dog into the delivery room to witness a medicated mother being put to sleep and her even sleepier baby being "delivered."

"The dog would get sick!" explains Dr. Bradley.

Other husbands object to their exclusion from the delivery room for more practical reasons.

"Perhaps they won't let me in the delivery room because they don't want me to realize how simple it is to deliver a baby," thinks this man. ". . . and if that's true, why should I pay $1,000 for something our ancestors did themselves?"

Whatever their reasons for secluding the wife and her obstetrician behind the closed doors of the delivery room, hospitals will sometimes go to bizarre lengths to protect their prerogatives. When a young college student in Arcata, California was told to leave his wife when she was in labor, he chained himself to her bed. Proclaiming his determination to remain by his wife's side throughout the birth of their first baby, John Quinn refused to budge.

"I love my wife," said Mr. Quinn, "and I feel it's my moral right as a husband and father to be there."

Unfortunately, the hospital did not agree. They called

the police, who forcibly removed the young man from his own wife's bedside.

Elisabeth Bing, the Berlin-born physiotherapist who popularized the Lamaze method of childbirth in the United States, also asserts that the husband has a clear-cut right to be with his wife during the birth of their baby. She points out that in a healthy marriage, the husband ought to be the dominant partner. As such, he needs definite scope to exercise his directive role when the child is born. In ideal circumstances, the husband must be able to both supervise and support his wife during labor. This may sound quite contradictory, but from personal experience I must agree that this is how things should be during childbirth. The husband ought to help his wife get through her labor by rubbing her back and providing reassurance, but he also ought to direct her through it. He may have to help her to change position even though she might be afraid to move, for example. Or he may have to remind her how to breathe, should she forget. Unfortunately, even when they admit him to the labor room, many hospitals see the husband as only a sort of "hand-holder." The obstetrician and hospital staff continue to direct the birth, thus robbing the couple of an experience in cooperation which should rightfully be theirs alone.

Although many people still look upon the husband's presence as an unnecessary "frill," he can literally make or break his wife's birth experience. One account of a natural birth describes a nurse's refusal to let the husband stay with his wife while she was being "prepped." By the time he was allowed to rejoin her, the labor pains had become so severe that the wife wanted a shot to relieve them.

"She was an electric knot, twisting and gasping and doubling up like in the movies," said the husband. Seeing that his wife was on the verge of losing control, he quickly began the Lamaze techniques to help her relax. Rubbing her back, giving her ice chips to suck on, and helping her breathe correctly, the husband completely involved himself with helping his wife get through labor.

"Nonny slowly regained control in direct proportion to her degree of relaxation," he remembered.

The baby was born about two hours later; a lighthearted atmosphere prevailed in the delivery room. Afterward, the couple remarked upon how much they had complemented and truly depended upon one another.[10]

From the wife's point of view, too, it's better if her husband leads her through childbirth. During the early years of marriage, she has gotten to know and trust her husband. By the time the first baby arrives, the wife has probably developed a certain amount of faith in her husband's dependability during times of crises. On the other hand, a woman may not even know the doctor who delivers her baby. Although it may be an obstetrician whom she has visited regularly, she does not usually have enough prior experience with this man to know whether he will be reliable enough to depend upon when she is unable to help herself. Doctors sometimes administer anesthesia, strip membranes, break the bag of waters, give injections, and perform rectal examinations without prior warning. Prenatal office visits don't provide a pregnant woman the opportunity to find out whether her obstetrician will be likely to do these things during the actual delivery, either.

Some women, who never before considered childbirth at home now say they don't want to be delivered by an obstetrician who also performs abortions. They wonder how a hospital can spend thousands of dollars to provide specialized care for premature babies weighing less than two pounds, while aborting other infants who weigh more and have a greater chance of survival.

"A hospital that does abortions leaves itself open for question as to the ethical and human kindness treatment it would give a maternity case," states one such mother. She plans to have her next baby at home.

From the husband's point of view, things were much easier in our grandparents' day; then the husband comforted his wife throughout labor and delivery. He also took care of many of the physical preparations for the impending birth and acted as host to the birth attendants. Clearly, it was then the mission of the doctor to *assist* at a birth, rather than to put a panic-stricken woman to sleep and *deliver* her of her limp, drug-laden baby. Both emotionally and in some ways medically, this was a more comfortable, workable mode of childbirth for the whole family.

When the delivery scene shifted to the hospital, though, these husband-wife-attendant relationships rapidly became distorted. Instead of the couple's calling upon the professionals for assistance, the obstetrician now tells the family when to go to the hospital, and sometimes even which hospital to go to. Once labor has begun, in fact, "everyone would prefer that the husband deposit (his wife) on the doorstep of the hospital and not return until she has had time to get over the effects of drugs and manipulations and has her hair combed and her prettiest nightgown on."[11]

While the banished husband chain-smokes in a waiting room, how is his wife getting along? The following chapter will examine her situation from the woman's point of view. For now, however, let's consider her labor objectively. Displaced from her bed at home, where she once could give birth in comfortable, secure surroundings, the mother-to-be is left alone in a narrow, high bed with adjustable cribside railings. Separated from her husband, her former source of protection against unwarranted intrusions, the anxious wife now finds herself isolated. From time to time, impersonal, white-uniformed strangers rush in to check on her progress. No matter how well-intentioned these people are, they are not involved with the mother in any deep way; they are neither family nor friends. How surprising is it, then, that in such alien surroundings the normal contractions of labor, so routine and bearable at home, seem like severe pains?

In a 1973 article in *Esquire*, Barbara Grizutti Harrison described how her treatment before her first child's birth robbed her of all vestiges of self-control.

"For most of the time, I was alone and frightened. . . . In rare moments of lucidity, I called—yelled—for the doctor. I groaned. I writhed. For eighteen hours, I screamed."[12]

Alone, thirsty, and badly frightened by the increasing intensity of her contractions, Mrs. Harrison represented an all-too-accurate picture of an average American woman in labor on one of our conventional maternity wards.

Could Mrs. Harrison have exaggerated her hospital experiences in order to write a more interesting story? For added objectivity, let's look at some reports on American hospital delivery from private patients who gave birth in Manhattan during the 1960s.

> I was screaming for Dr. M. because I had excruciating pain.
>
> The resident came in. I was appalled at the complete lack of manners. . . . They just stick a finger up you, treat you like a cow, an animal.
>
> I kept calling for my doctor, and I didn't react the way they wanted . . . And the nurses kept yelling at me.
>
> The intern was a sadistic little squirt.
>
> Some of these nurses are so hostile . . . the way they press your abdomen, the manner of shaving, very fast and very hard.
>
> I remember being very annoyed with the nurse and the doctor, because they made me feel very guilty for having pain.[13]

In what would probably be regarded by these women as a masterpiece of understatement, obstetrician Herbert Thoms explains that "the total effect of an unpleasant environment on an anxious and uninformed woman is not very conducive to a happy childbirth experience." Citing the unfamiliar, austere surroundings of the hospital and the lack of personalized attention to the needs of the patient, Dr. Thoms concludes that for childbirth, "shifting the scene to the hospital, in spite of increased safety, has in other ways made the expectant mother more apprehensive."

Forced Labor, a sociological study of maternity care in the United States by Nancy Stoller Shaw, places much of the blame for our sub-human treatment of childbirth on the hospital setting. Because the hospital staff and maternity patients have fundamentally different needs (which often oppose each other), the birth can't conveniently be treated as a beautiful family event. So, to make labor as easy as possible for the doctors and nurses, the patient is "isolated, stripped, emptied, drugged, immobilized, and 'delivered' within the protective walls of the hospital."[14]

Many critics of childbirth at home say that the answer to the current impasse lies in "humanizing the hospitals." Yet *Forced Labor* points out that the hospital is medical territory. Even if a woman's husband can go with her, the balance of power shifts to the hospital once the wife is admitted as a patient. Laymen are not familiar with the hospital's hierarchy, geography, treatments and terminology. So they are usually awed and intimidated. Consequently, they are in a poor position to challenge the hospital's procedures, no matter how "patently inaccurate, degrading, or unnecessary" they seem.[15]

In *Understanding Natural Childbirth,* writing about the alien hospital environment, Dr. Herbert Thoms pointed out that the maternity ward setting and procedures often increased the mother's fear of childbirth.

"Furthermore," he added, "intense emotional stress, especially anxiety and fear, can be highly unfavorable to the childbirth process."

Dr. Thoms made this observation in 1950. Twenty-five years later, however, few obstetricians seem to accept or even understand it. Although a 1974 book on childbirth admits that birth may be "more protracted, difficult, painful and dangerous if the mother is fearful,"[16] most doctors seem reluctant to take any meaningful steps to reduce her anxiety in the hospital.

What effect does stress actually have upon the mother and upon her unborn baby? In order to answer this question, we have to look at exactly what happens to mothers whose labors are disturbed.

Dr. Robert A. Bradley, author of *Husband-Coached Childbirth*, is one obstetrician who's an authority on interruptions during labor. He explains that even to his patients, who are trained in natural-childbirth techniques of relaxation, his "occasional vaginal examinations to determine the dilation of the cervix constitute rather rude interruptions which momentarily disrupt the smooth working pattern of the process." Dr. Bradley started using husbands as coaches after he noticed that his patients could remain calm and relaxed during contractions only when their husbands were by their sides. If the men left the room—even for just a few moments—their wives' labors were adversely affected. Without the husbands, the women immediately became anxious, tense, and unable to relax. As a result, their contractions quickly began to feel painful.

Other obstetricians have noted that labor frequently slows down when the mother travels from her home to the hospital, and later when she must move from the labor-room bed to the delivery table. This is not uncommon, but most women don't expect it, so they are likely to become anxious. A mother whose contractions suddenly seem to evaporate has every right to feel confused and distressed. Unfortunately, her self-confidence often erodes further when ignorant hospital attendants make her feel that she has somehow stopped her contractions on purpose.

"Come on," they may tell her. "You're wasting our time."

Recent research on labor patterns in animals has provided information that could shed light upon this disturbing phenomenon. An article in *Science* reported that when researchers picked up mice during their deliveries, the mice who were thus interrupted took twenty minutes to deliver their next babies. (An undisturbed mother mouse would only take twelve minutes.) Moving a pregnant mouse during labor, before any of her babies were born, resulted in a delay of four hours for the delivery of the entire litter. A four-hour wait doesn't sound very long—until we realize that in a human mother this delay would equal fifty-six hours!

Other experiments have shown the price which might be paid for such delayed labors. Mice who suffer stress during labor have more stillbirths; the fear which tightens their muscles and constricts their blood vessels decreases the blood (and oxygen) supply to the fetus. Could this happen to humans? Of course. But obstetrical interference usually produces a live baby. The point is, both forceps and Caesarean deliveries pose added risks to mothers and babies. If births could take place in a relaxed atmosphere, far less obstetrical intervention would be necessary.

Quiet, undisturbed surroundings during labor have always been considered absolutely important by animal breeders and veterinarians. Researchers working under Dr. Harry F. Harlow at the University of Wisconsin's primate laboratories discovered this the hard way, though. Their assignment was to separate infant monkeys from their mothers immediately after birth, for Dr. Harlow's study of mother-child relationships in rhesus monkeys. Whenever a staff worker tried to remain in the room during the birth, however, the mother monkey's contractions would "become irregular and even cease because of the emotional disturbance created by the presence of the human intruder."[17] As a result, the researchers had to wait outside until the birth was all over.

Mice and monkeys are not the only mammals which react adversely to disturbances during labor. When female dogs receive emotionally distressing stimuli during labor, their contractions are inhibited and their deliveries delayed, according to an article in the *American Journal of Obstetrics and Gynecology*.

"The adrenalin triggered by the autonomic nervous system in response to stress actually inhibits the release of the chemical oxytocin," claims Helen Wessel. Her book, *Natural Childbirth and the Family*, explains how oxytocin, a hormone released from the mother's pituitary gland, makes the uterus contract during labor. Biochemists believe oxytocin also releases milk when the mother nurses her baby. This would explain why anxiety in the mother decreases her supply of milk. As most farmers know, an earthquake, or sometimes even a storm, stops cows from giving milk for up to three days. And when a mother gives birth in a hospital where she feels insecure, she may not be able to nurse her baby for as long as nine days.[18]

"If disturbing a mother's emotions in labor so drastically affected uterine action in rhesus monkeys, could this be true also for human mothers?"

Dr. Bradley posed this question in 1955, discussing the value of undisturbed conditions for an ideal, peaceful childbirth atmosphere. He admitted, however, that such conditions could hardly be achieved in any hospital delivery room. In fact, said he, they are "most nearly met by the environment of a mother's bedroom in her own home and the reassuring nearness of familiar and loved faces rather than those of strangers."

Despite the logic of these arguments, the overwhelming majority of American obstetricians still continue to insist that all their patients have their babies in the hospital. Why? According to anthropologist Ashley Montagu, the single, most compelling reason that obstetricians insist on hospital deliveries is that they are more convenient for the doctor. Of course, few obstetricians would be willing to admit this so candidly. Instead, they would probably dwell on the belief that the hospital is the only place safe enough for childbirth.

But is it? Recent evidence suggests that the hospital's equipment, environment, personnel, and procedures not only fail
to guarantee a safe delivery, but may even serve to make it
more hazardous. The next two chapters explore this assertion
logically, for only a thoughtful examination of the pros and
cons can help parents reach a solid decision on whether their
baby ought to be born in a hospital or at home.

Before going into this question, however, it might be
helpful to scrutinize our general conviction that births *should*
take place in the hospital. Why have Americans in particular
been so unquestioning in holding this assumption?

Fully 98 percent of the people now alive were born at
home. In some societies, birth is considered a pleasant social
affair, according to anthropologist Margaret Mead. Pediatrician T. Berry Brazelton tells of witnessing a young girl's first
delivery in Mexico, along with some twenty to thirty of her
family and friends. This concerned, involved group, which
included the babies and children of the family, made up a
moral-support section for the young mother-to-be. They
cheered her on through the entire labor and birth.

Even in this country, the custom in the early part of this
century called for the wife's husband to be present, to provide
reassurance, and to assist the midwife in a variety of ways. In
fact, home births were prevalent prior to about 1940. Before
about 1900, hospitals were wisely avoided by the majority of
American women, due to their poor safety record. "Unless
they were on their deathbeds, women refused to go to the
hospital, because to do so meant almost surely to contract
childbed fever."[19]

When Ignaz Semmelweiss discovered that obstetricians
could prevent childbed fever by washing their hands between
handling cadavers and attending expectant mothers, the way
was cleared for hospital delivery to become more widespread.
Doctors began urging all their obstetrical patients to come to
the hospital for childbirth, since this would make it easier for
them to see more patients in less time. It would also insure that

obstetricians had access to whatever equipment they needed to assist the small minority of mothers who suffered real complications. In this way American women were persuaded to deliver in the hospital for extrinsic reasons. That is, the normal woman went to the hospital not because it was proved to be better for *her* or for *her baby*, but because it was better for her obstetrician and for the few mothers who presented complications.

This trend illustrates a concept that is well understood by psychologists and anthropologists, but relatively unsuspected by the general public . . . "methods and procedures of childbirth . . . are products of historical and cultural factors, influenced by scientific and social trends. *The childbirth situation is in no way absolute or permanent.*"[20] (Italics mine)

Awareness of this fact is gradually dawning upon the American consciousness. In an era of growing desire for both consumer and feminine rights, American women are beginning to demand more control over their own deliveries. As Constance A. Bean explains in *Methods of Childbirth*, "consumers have become more knowledgeable about health care and institutional care in general. They are less tolerant of frustrations than they used to be." This trend, although a healthy one, can give rise to paradoxical situations. More and more young couples, well-read and well-prepared for childbirth by prenatal classes, encounter doctor and hospital resistance to the kind of birth experience they desire. The results can be compared to the irresistible force when it meets the immovable object. Disillusioned and bitter, these young parents-to-be must choose between sacrificing their natural childbirth ideals and dropping out of the medical care system completely. This is just what happened to my husband and me. We chose home childbirth only after exhausting every possible avenue of compromise with the medical establishment.

Soon we discovered that we were not alone. Almost without exception, a group of middle-class parents who had their

babies at home in the early 1970s did so because they had
arrived at the same impasse. Like us, most of them had gone to
the hospital for the births of their first children. Like us, they
felt unable to return to repeat an experience which many
thought would be dangerous for the mothers and for their
babies, too.

"Degrading, discouraging, and even downright distasteful," said a Salt Lake City registered nurse, when talking about
her maternity stay at a prominent institution.

She persuaded her husband to agree to home birth for
their fourth baby. Its successful home delivery confirmed her
suspicion that the "pain and complications of labor and delivery are to a great extent generated in the hospital environment."

Other women who were interviewed described their hospitals as factories and complained about the coldness of their
staffs. Most of these wives had strongly resented being ordered around. They had been prepared to play an *active* part
in their deliveries and were not prepared to accept the *passive*
role which the nurses and doctors expected their "good patients" to adopt.

The couples described their unattended home births as
delightful, exhilarating, satisfying and spiritually ennobling.
In fact, one Illinois mother, who had been traumatized and
suffered massive hemorrhages after the hospital births of her
first two children, delivered her next two babies at home with
absolutely no complications.

Due to our cultural conditioning, most Americans would
probably be shocked that this mother could take such a
"foolish" chance. Yet a group of Northern California obstetricians who perform home deliveries agree that panic can ag-
gravate, or even cause excessive postpartum bleeding.[21]
Would panic not be more likely to strike the patients who are
strapped down in a noisy hospital delivery room, frightened
and weakened by lonely hours of pain? Many people think
panic would be far less likely to occur in the women who give
birth naturally in their own quiet bedrooms at home.

A 1971 book on the psychological experience of childbirth explains why so many of the girls of California's counterculture seem "willing to give up a measure of safety for the mother in order to avoid the strange hospital environment and alien medical authority."[22] Once again, previous maternity ward experiences often left the young parents overflowing with impotent rage. Due to their particular concern with natural, organic modes of being, couples like this feel especially reluctant to delegate their deliveries to institutions that insist on treating childbirth as if it were surgery.

Do hospitals really view the pregnant woman as a surgical patient? The following chapter describes what happens to the young mother during her stay on a typical American maternity ward.

NOTES

1. Jean McCann, "They Want to Have Their Babies at Home," *Marriage*, June 1971, p. 14.
2. Deborah Schwabach, "I Had My Baby in My Bedroom," *Redbook*, October 1968, p. 15.
3. Orde Coombs, "Some Babies Have to Be Born Twice," *Redbook*, October 1972, p. 77.
4. Constance A. Bean, *Methods of Childbirth* (Garden City, N.Y.: Doubleday & Company, 1972), p. 191.
5. The Boston Women's Health Book Collective, *Our Bodies, Ourselves* (New York: Simon & Schuster, 1971), p. 238.
6. Elliott H. McCleary, *New Miracles of Childbirth* (New York: David McKay, 1974), p. 154.
7. H.M.I. Liley, M.D., and Beth Day, *Modern Motherhood* (New York: Random House, 1965), p. 62.
8. Deborah Tanzer and Jean L. Block, *Why Natural Childbirth?* (Garden City, N.Y.: Doubleday & Company, 1972), p. 168.
9. Ibid., p. 216.
10. Donna and Rodger Ewy, *Preparation for Childbirth* (Boulder, Colorado: Pruett Publishing Co., 1970), p. 103.
11. Lester Dessez Hazell, *Commonsense Childbirth* (New York: G.P. Putnam's Sons, 1969), p. xxxii.

12. Barbara Grizutti Harrison, "Men Don't Know Nothin' 'Bout Birthin' Babies," *Esquire*, July 1973, p. 133.
13. Deborah Tanzer and Jean L. Block, op. cit., pp. 100-102.
14. Nancy Stoller Shaw, *Forced Labor: Maternity Care in the United States* (Elmsford, N.Y.: Pergamon Press, 1974), p. 134.
15. Ibid., p. 135.
16. Elliott H. McCleary, op. cit., p. 225.
17. Robert A. Bradley, M.D., *Husband-Coached Childbirth* (New York: Harper & Row, 1965), p. 23.
18. Gladys West Hendrick, *My First 300 Babies* (Pasadena, California: My First 300 Babies, 1964), p. 148.
19. Lester Dessez Hazell, op. cit., p. xxviii.
20. Deborah Tanzer and Jean L. Block, op. cit., p. 2.
21. Ellen Sander, "Childbirth at Home," *Mademoiselle*, May 1972, p. 204.
22. Arthur and Libby Colman, *Pregnancy: the Psychological Experience* (New York: Herder & Herder, 1971), p. 91.

OTHER SOURCES
(listed as they appear in text)

Elisabeth Bing, *The Adventure of Birth* (New York: Simon & Schuster, 1970), p. 9.
Herbert Thoms, M.D., *Understanding Natural Childbirth* (New York: McGraw-Hill Book Company, 1950), p. 13.
Boston Children's Medical Center, *Pregnancy, Birth and the Newborn Baby* (Boston: Boston Children's Medical Center, 1971).
Ashley Montagu, appearing on *The Tonight Show*, November 16, 1973, interviewed by Johnny Carson on NBC.
T. Berry Brazelton, M.D., "What Childbirth Drugs Can Do to Your Child," *Redbook*, February 1971, p. 65.
Shirley Anthony, in a letter appearing in the Reader Reaction columns of *California Living*. (San Francisco: The magazine of the *San Francisco Sunday Examiner* and *Chronicle*, December 8, 1974).

2

THE AMERICAN WAY OF BIRTH

"While the hospital delivery may have offered a partial solution for medical and surgical emergencies, to process the vast majority of women who present no such problems through such routine has wrought all kinds of havoc on the social order of our family life." For this reason, the president of the International Childbirth Education Association argued that American-style delivery harms family unity. Indeed our current birth customs obviously do divide, rather than unite the family. Such damage to the family unit seems even more obnoxious when we realize that the birth of a baby is one of the family's biggest milestones.

The damage done to family life by our conventional way of childbirth begins when the mother must leave her home. If labor starts at night, she must rouse herself, dress, and pack her belongings between contractions. Then she must undertake the uncomfortable trip to the hospital.

Even if the mother's labor proceeds normally, the effects of rough, bumpy roads, or sudden maneuvers in traffic feel traumatic. A woman in labor can suffer physical damage from bad roads; there is also no way she can get comfortable in a car. The anxiety she must feel every time the car screeches to a stop or swerves around a corner can only serve to increase her overall tension. The more tense she becomes, the more likely she will experience her contractions as painful. On the other hand, the journey may make her contractions less regular and less effective. Either way, the trip to the hospital interferes with the smooth progress of a normal labor.

After reaching the hospital, the couple must find an entrance that's open—not always an easy job in the middle of the night, especially if it's raining! They must be prepared to pay a deposit of several hundred dollars, unless they carry medical insurance. (Fortunately, we didn't have to confront this financial hurdle, since I was entitled to free care in a military hospital.)

To us, it was the admission form which presented some difficulty. It seemed decidedly weighted in favor of the doctor and the hospital. Admission consent was worded in such a way that by signing into the hospital, the patient also gave permission for any tests, drugs, and anesthetics to be administered.

I was quite upset when I read this form. My idea of how childbirth should be didn't include any of these items! Finally, I solved the problem by crossing out several lines of the statement, inserting my own wishes above the signature. I wrote that I did not want an episiotomy, anesthetic, or any more drugs than were absolutely necessary. The doctors didn't react very well when they saw it, but it worked. As far as I know, I was the only maternity patient on the ward who did not receive a routine episiotomy, spinal anesthetic, or any of the other procedures which were standard at the time.

Once the average woman is officially accepted into the hospital, what happens next? After saying good-bye to her husband, she must go to a labor room, give all her own clothes to the nurse, and don a short hospital shirt. If the doctor confirms that she is really in labor, she will be "prepped." This term, borrowed from surgical jargon, refers to the preparation of the area to be cut. In a maternity patient, the incision site is the perineum. Accordingly, the mother's entire pubic area—from her navel to her rectum—is shaved and then painted or sprayed with disinfectant. This delicate operation, often hastily performed by an inexperienced nurse, can frighten even a prepared woman. It can be dangerous, too. In *The Female Eunuch*, Germaine Greer describes how a rushed nurse almost cut off her clitoris while performing this shave. Even when the mother gets through the experience with all her vital parts intact, the shave is demeaning and causes needless embarrassment, tension and resentment.

Why do most doctors insist that their obstetrical patients be prepped as if they are about to undergo surgery? Most frequently they say it's more sanitary. But doctors who have tried omitting the shave report no increase of infection—even after thousands of deliveries without it.[1]

Another reason some obstetricians give for shaving is that it makes it easier to perform an episiotomy. Yet "no hair grows where the incision should be," according to *Commonsense Childbirth*. As one irreverent doctor puts it, shaving the perineum in order to do an episiotomy makes as much sense as shaving a man's moustache in order to perform a tonsillectomy!

Besides the anxiety and embarrassment associated with the prep, women who have undergone the procedure before dread the soreness and itching they will face when the pubic hair begins to grow in again. Small boils often occur in the disturbed hair follicles, and infections can result from the nicks made by the hospital's razor. When these annoyances join with the soreness and pulling of stitches in the episiotomy, the total discomfort can practically drive a new mother up the wall.

Fortunately, some hospitals are beginning to modify their regulations on the shave; the pubic hair can easily be clipped close enough so the doctor can see what he is doing. But the majority of hospitals still insist upon giving a routine enema to all their maternity patients. The reason for this is to evacuate the lower bowel and give the baby more room to descend through the birth canal. While the intention is laudable, is the trauma worth it? Many young mothers describe the enema—often the first they ever received—as more painful than the birth itself. Frequently, mothers have accused the enema of being the single factor which changed their contractions from being quite bearable to acutely agonizing. These are some of their comments:

> I was more afraid of the enema than the birth. I tried to get out of it by not eating too much.

> Then the woman came in and gave me an enema and I wish they had told me about this. It was very distressing to me.

> They prepped me and I think one of the worst experiences is to have a contraction when you're having an enema.

> They prepared me, and gave me an enema, which was just awful. The enema was worse than. . . it was terrible. It gave me terrible cramps.

> I've had enemas before, but this time being pregnant, with all this pressure on my stomach, and all this water in me, I just felt like I was going to explode.[2]

A few doctors now think predelivery enemas should only be given if absolutely necessary. A 1962 article in the *American Journal of Obstetrics and Gynecology* told why:

> The physician who is not present during the administration of the enema is usually unaware of the patient's discomfort and even embarrassment during this procedure. . . . The soapsuds enema has disadvantages in addition to the patient's discomfort. It is irritating to the mucosa. . . . Side effects caused by general discomfort, mild or marked cramps, and rectal irritation amounted to 84.8 percent. . . .

Besides receiving an enema, which produces such painful stimuli around the perineum, the mother will be subjected to repeated rectal and vaginal examinations. Their purpose is to determine how labor is progressing so the doctor can time his arrival to anticipate the impending birth. A considerate attendant will explain why these manipulations are necessary, but mothers still dread these annoying, often painful interruptions. One woman told me that the worst parts of her labor were the times when a young intern monitored her contractions with his gloved finger completely inserted in her rectum, which was still very sore from the enema. Incidents like this help explain why such a large percentage of American mothers "complain bitterly of the depersonalized way in which they [are] handled by doctors they [have] never seen before."[3]

Probably the most discouraging aspect of labor, however, is the separation of the wife from her husband and her subsequent isolation. Typically, she may spend an entire day alone, except for brief visits from the staff to check on her condition. This loneliness of the laboring mother is practically unique in our country. Anthropologist Margaret Mead reports that no primitive society leaves a mother alone during labor, and to turn her over to strangers would be abolutely unthinkable.[4]

> The interval of time between the prep and the onset of second [or pushing] stage is usually a lonely and bewildering time. Most women are not prepared for the fact that the end of first [cervical dilation] stage, not the delivery, is the hardest part of labor. The symptoms that this part of labor brings are frightening to those who do not expect them, and loneliness and pain often become unbearable. At the same time this part of labor does not excite much activity on the part of the staff, so the laboring woman often feels that she is abandoned and that her labor is not progressing adequately.[5]

Prior to this, pain-relieving drugs are usually given to the mother (whether she wants them or not!). Out of all the analgesics, or pain-killing drugs, Demerol seems to be the current favorite with American obstetricians. A synthetic version of morphine, Demerol has to be given at least several hours before childbirth. Otherwise, the baby will be born with too high a level of depressant in its bloodstream. If the baby is born too soon after the mother receives a full dose of Demerol, respiratory equipment will probably be required to force the newborn infant to start breathing.[6]

Since Demerol poses such a risk to the baby, its pain-killing effects must be quite amazing, right? *Wrong!* For years, mothers have been reporting that it is woefully inadequate as an analgesic. Women who were prepared for natural childbirth and took Demerol said that it did "nothing to relieve powerful contractions."[7] Instead, it interfered with their ability to relax. In fact, most patients who have taken Lamaze childbirth classes try to avoid taking Demerol. They know it will destroy their powers of concentration and make them feel like drunks trying to walk a straight line.

In an article in *Today's Health,* one mother gave this opinion about Demerol's effect on her labor:

> The Demerol that accompanied my first childbirth distorted my time sense, sweeping me along in a current that had no exit. Bottomless. It did not kill the pain but trapped me inside it, and I can still remember the anguish of that helpless drifting.[8]

The drug that causes the most severe disorientation in mothers, however, is scopolamine. Similar to LSD in structure, "scope" makes the woman so restless during contractions that she loses self-control and becomes unable to cooperate. Under the influence of scopolamine, the patient may tear off her clothes, swear at the nurses, or resort to violence. Dr. Robert Bradley aptly describes these mothers in labor as "wild-eyed medicated maniacs, all conscious control long gone via medication."

Because of these disturbing effects of "scope," women who receive it must be physically restrained.

"There are hospitals not far from New York City where patients with football helmets on them are put in padded beds 'scoped to the eyeballs,'" reported obstetrician William J. Sweeney in *Woman's Doctor*. Dr. Sweeney's book is not a romantic novel; it describes American obstetrics in the 1970s.

Sometimes the nurses must forcibly prevent a "scoped" woman from getting out of bed; then the patient may think she is being attacked. It's up to the nurses and orderlies to restrain her so she won't harm herself or jeopardize her baby's safety.

"Scope makes it difficult to give anything but a custodial type of care," reports one nurse. She explains that the routine use of the drug complicates the job of labor-room attendants. The nurses have a hard time treating "scoped" women like competent human beings. For this reason, many excellent nurses try to avoid maternity duty. As a result, mothers in labor are deprived of the support they would otherwise receive from the best nursing care.

Mothers often suffer more than they need to because of scope. One of its most distressing side effects has been to deny analgesic help for labor. Women under the influence of scope may become so irrational that the nurses can't recognize their legitimate requests for pain relief. They may conclude that the patient's cries for help are caused by her scope-induced hallucinations instead of by her labor pains.[9] Once more, the mother ends up the loser.

It seems incredible that the consumer should have to endure such bizarre side effects from a drug that does not even relieve her pain. But scopolamine has no analgesic properties; it's an amnesic, or "forgetfulness" drug. Like its chemical cousin LSD, scope acts upon the mind; it changes thought patterns in such a way that memory is destroyed. In doing this, scope can also cause the hallucinations which make the affected mothers behave so unpredictably.

Most of the recent books on pregnancy and birth (written for the expectant mother) don't bother to discuss these serious effects of scopolamine. Instead, one of them tells the mother that "modern chemical technology has made it possible for labor to be a comfortable experience."[10]

Since scopolamine has so many disadvantages, why do doctors continue to order it for women in labor? According to *Forced Labor*, it's because the use of this amnesiac makes things easier for the hospital staff. Once a mother has been "scoped," the nurses "need not worry about spending too much time on amenities, emotional support, conversation, or modesty protection."[11]

Even if the mother has decided she wants to be awake for the birth of her baby, and even if she remains calm and cooperative during labor, scope may be administered—as long as she gave permission for anesthesia at her first prenatal appointment.

> The agreement seven months ago to "sleep" can be used to justify scopolamine administration even though the patients are *never* told they are getting amnesiacs instead of anesthesia. Even when the woman does not *want* to be asleep, the permission is there.[12]

Although Demerol and scopolamine are the most commonly used, there are several other powerful drugs which may be given during labor. Barbiturates such as Seconal can put the mother to sleep, while a labor-stimulating oxytocic hormone speeds up her contractions. *Commonsense Childbirth* says that doctors often give such chemical agents when labor slows down, even though they are aware of the dangers of a precipitate birth. In *Our Bodies, Ourselves,* a young mother tells how she was treated with these drugs.

> At the hospital I got some injections of what I thought was Pitocin. My labor was very intense and unexpectedly short—four hours. . . . My daughter had to be delivered by forceps because her heartbeat was slowing down

and I couldn't push her out quickly enough. I was told
her life had been endangered because my contractions
were too strong.
. . . It turned out that I had gotten Pitocin to induce
my labor for a time, then Demerol to slow my contractions down, because they were going too fast.
Now that I look back, I think that perhaps the Pitocin
stimulated my labor too strongly so that indeed it wasn't
natural, and was even dangerous . . .

This mother's suspicions have been proven correct. A
recent study revealed that one out of four infants whose
mothers received oxytocic drugs suffered from lack of oxygen. When the mother received both oxytocin *and* regional
anesthesia, the number of endangered unborn infants rose to
50 percent.[13] (In the laboratory, oxytocin and anesthesia
given to female monkeys during labor have produced brain
damage, including cerebral palsy, in their fetuses.)

Besides stimulating labor once it has begun, oxytocic
drugs can also be used to artificially induce the birth of a baby.
According to *Lancet,* a British medical journal, more than half
of all English births in hospitals are now artificially induced.
Raymond Booth, secretary of the Royal College of Obstetricians and Gynaecologists, agrees that this practice subjects
some mothers and their babies to needless risks.

Why are so many British women asked to have their
babies by appointment? The National Childbirth Trust claims
it's because staff members of maternity units want to be able to
close the ward and take time off![14]

In this country, too, the trend is toward more inductions.
According to *Immaculate Deception: A New Look at Women and
Childbirth in America,* "induced labor is so common today that it
is routine in many American hospitals. . . ."[15] These inductions take place despite the fact that most obstetricians agree
they are more dangerous than waiting for labor to begin by
itself.

Dr. Roberto Caldeyro-Barcia, who heads the International Federation of Gynecologists and Obstetricians, warns

that when labor is induced with oxytocic hormones, almost 75 percent of the mother's uterine contractions are so strong that they reduce the amount of oxygen reaching the baby's brain. In a study he supervised at twelve Latin American medical centers, Dr. Caldeyro-Barcia discovered that the forceful contractions of induced labor frequently caused disalignment of certain bones in the infant's skull. This disalignment of the parietal bones occurred twice as often in induced labors as in normal labors. Not only does the deformation elongate the infant's head, it can also cause "damage to the infant brain, possible hemorrhage inside the brain, and signs of asphyxia and cerebral trauma."[16]

The use of drugs which stimulate contractions artificially is a perfect example of the way our American way of birth has become so perverted that stumbling blocks are actually put in the way of nature. "With each additional stumbling block we add a pharmacological or instrumental detour and in the process become further and further removed from that orderly precision which is normal labor. . . . Thus the very tools which should be lifesaving become damage-dealing instead."[17]

A good example of a lifesaving tool which causes damage when used for normal childbirth is anesthesia. Certainly, the discovery of ether and chloroform in the last century made it possible for doctors to intervene more effectively in obstructed labors. "Twilight sleep" was introduced by 1907, and it quickly became popular throughout most of the civilized world. This morphine-scopolamine combination enabled every mother to undergo labor in a dreamy, narcotized condition. Since her trancelike state made it more difficult to deliver the baby unaided, however, even the normal mothers soon needed obstetrical assistance. Naturally, this development did a lot to help move the locale of birth from the home to the hospital.

Once again, sociological rather than purely medical reasons contribute to the formation of childbirth mores.

Awake and Aware points out the connection between certain anesthetic discoveries and the growing demand for women's rights in the early years of this century.

> Had chloroform and twilight sleep come into the world at a different time, it is doubtful if women would have accepted them so readily. In their eagerness to liberate themselves from civil and social oppression, women easily accepted what they considered liberation from their biological oppression. . . . Perhaps they would have chosen to *experience* their biological destiny if they had already achieved what they considered to be their social, political and economic destiny.[18]

Mothers who had children under such anesthesia often carry very unpleasant memories of the births.

"I felt like I was dying," reports one lady.

"You feel like you're falling into a whirlpool," said another patient. "You get dizzy and extremely nauseous."

After about fifty years, obstetricians began to realize that for a normal birth, the dangers of general anesthesia far outweighed its benefits. Anesthesia can slow the heartbeat, depress breathing, and slacken the flow of blood through the mother's body, which decreases the oxygen reaching the baby. General anesthesia frequently causes violent vomiting; since the mother is asleep, she may breathe the regurgitated matter into her lungs. According to one source, the complications that follow—asphyxiation, pneumonia, etc.—are still the greatest cause of maternal deaths in the United States.[19]

We are still, in fact, discovering the harmful consequences of anesthesia. Recently, a Stanford University research team discovered that women who worked in operating rooms where they inhaled the vapors of anesthetic gases had miscarriages three times more than normal. Out of thirty-six nurses who worked in the operating room and became pregnant, ten lost their babies. Of thirty-seven female anesthetists, fourteen miscarried, whereas only six out of fifty-eight other women doctors were unable to carry their babies to term.[20]

Similar studies in England and Denmark came to the same conclusions about the high incidence of miscarriages in women who were exposed to anesthetic gases. The British study, which covered 80 percent of all their women anesthetists, also discovered that these women had a higher percentage of abnormal babies than did the population at large.

Because of all the risks associated with general anesthesia, it has largely been replaced by a variety of regional substances, sometimes referred to as conduction anesthesia. "Regionals" are drugs which paralyze the nerves. Spinals and saddle blocks are two popular types of regional anesthesia; a spinal will stop the patient from feeling any sensation below the waist; saddle blocks numb only the area where she sits down.

Each regional anesthetic carries its own particular risk. A spinal must be administered by an extremely skillful anesthesiologist because it calls for the injection of the anesthetic into the spinal fluid around the lower backbone. If the puncture is too large, spinal fluid can leak out of the spinal column, reducing the pressure around the cord and causing a severe, unremitting headache. Some experts estimate that one in five mothers suffer from postspinal headaches, with the pain being far worse than the birth pain the spinal was supposed to relieve. Other side effects which may be caused by spinals include leg paralysis, backaches, difficulty in urinating, weakness, and pain at the puncture.

Furthermore, according to *Pregnancy, Birth, and Family Planning*, spinals also stop labor! Therefore they can be used only for the actual birth. Given a choice, many women would prefer to endure the temporary pain of childbirth rather than suffer the often long-lasting effects of spinal anesthesia. The only trouble is, in many American hospitals, women have no choice.

It is clear that few if any women are told of the risks to themselves or their babies from particular drugs and anesthetics, particularly the most common ones that are used routinely in the majority of normal deliveries though not really necessary. Most often doctors have given them instead completely positive, glowing descriptions of the drugs' benefits.[21]

Other types of regionals include caudals, pudendals, epidurals and paracervical infiltrations. Each kind carries its own dangers and side effects. Unless a caudal is injected into exactly the right spot of the tailbone, for instance, all of the toxic drug may not reach the caudal canal. Whatever goes "astray" may cause a sudden drop in the mother's blood pressure; this results in oxygen deprivation for the baby, just when he needs oxygen most. According to neonatal expert Virginia Apgar, the normal birth process decreases the amount of oxygen that reaches the infant via the placenta. Another drastic drop in the baby's oxygen supply at this time can lead to brain injury or even death.

When an emergency like this occurs, the paralyzed mother can't push the baby out by herself; the doctor must cut open her perineum and drag the baby out with forceps. But these crucial operations bring additional risks. According to Dr. Apgar, both the use of forceps and the precipitate birth which may result under these circumstances can cause bleeding in the infant's brain. Margaret Mead aptly described this type of situation when she said, "The emphasis put upon the prevention of pain has . . . diverted attention from possible damaging consequences for the infant."

During the 1950s, as general anesthesia became less popular, "regionals" were hailed as completely safe. Doctors have learned since, however, that conduction anesthesia can cause spinal shock, meningitis, arachnoiditis (inflammation of the membranes of the spinal cord), and even cardiac arrest. Like general anesthetics, regionals quickly cross the placental barrier and enter the fetal bloodstream.[22] More recent studies indicate that "all regional anesthesia can prolong second-stage labor and result in an increased use of oxytocin and an increased incidence of forceps deliveries."[23]

What exactly are forceps? They are twin blades made out of curved surgical steel. They can be inserted into the mother's vagina, applied to the baby's head, and then locked. By bracing himself and pulling, the doctor can use the forceps to rotate the baby and extract it from the birth canal. When used by an experienced, skillful obstetrician, there is no doubt that forceps can be very helpful for the tiny minority of complicated births. Using them for routine deliveries, however, is questioned by many authorities.

Since the early part of this century, "American obstetricians have come to use forceps for most of their deliveries, even the uncomplicated ones."[24] Dr. Llewellyn-Jones, the author of *Everywoman and Her Body*, conservatively estimates that well over one-third of American infants are delivered with forceps. He ascribes this to the fact that "women in labour in America are very heavily sedated, and often are given an anesthetic so that they are unable to help in pushing the baby into the world."

Another study in Rochester, New York found that many impatient obstetricians use instruments when there is absolutely no medical need of them, thus causing premature delivery of the infants.[25] Only in America, it seems, has the safety of infants been subordinated to the demands of such "advanced" medical technology.

Every other country approaches the use of forceps much more cautiously. Holland, which usually has one of the world's lowest infant mortality rates, employs forceps for only 1.5 percent of births. When the need for obstetrical intervention arises, Dutch doctors prefer to use the vacuum extractor. They think it's safer for the baby, and use it for 2.5 percent of their deliveries.[26] (Vacuum extraction is also used in France and Spain. While it's very traumatic for the mother, it's believed to pose less risk than forceps to the baby.)

England, another country which has a low infant mortality rate, also uses forceps in only a small percentage of births. Most estimates place the figure at less than 5 percent. In Asia, only one percent of infants are delivered by forceps, and the U.S.S.R. uses forceps for a scant 2 percent of deliveries.

There can be no denying the fact that forceps save lives during a complicated birth. But no other country uses them for as many *normal* births as does the United States. Furthermore, their use requires extremely good judgment, caution, and skill.

In 1970, an intern, a resident and a third-year medical student performed a mid-forceps delivery at a teaching hospital in California. Although it had been anticipated as a normal delivery, the fetal heartbeat dropped to below 100 beats per minute during labor. This was a danger signal, so the baby was delivered with forceps as quickly as possible. Because of the forceps bruises, the infant couldn't open her eyes for three weeks. She was battered and swollen; brain damage lowered her I.Q. to about 15. Now she is a small child. She will probably never be able to talk or feed herself. Her life expectancy is about sixty years.

If such a delivery took place today at a perinatal center, a Caesarean section would probably be performed, according to Dr. Roger Freeman, obstetrics chief at the University of Southern California Medical School.

"You can drag a lot of things out through the pelvis with a forceps, but I don't think that's using good judgment," he says. "However," adds Dr. Freeman, "that's the way most of us were trained and that's the way obstetrics is practiced generally in America today."[27]

During an interview in 1974, one of the directors of the American Academy of husband-coached childbirth mentioned the vast numbers of children who suffer severe brain damage during forceps deliveries.

"They have a whole ward full of children who are institutionalized because the forceps used to pull them out of their mothers messed them up so badly," he reported.

An employee on one of these "forceps wards" at a state hospital was so affected by these pathetic victims of botched deliveries that he enrolled his wife in a husband-coached-childbirth class as soon as she became pregnant.

Supposedly, more recent graduates of medical schools learn to avoid the high forceps delivery used formerly. With this technique, forceps were used to reach high up into the birth canal, "requiring a good deal of force to extract the baby."[28] (Excessive traction with forceps, with a resulting stretching of the infant's neck, has been mentioned as one of the suspected causes of birth-connected cerebral palsy.)

Lately, the low forceps delivery has become more popular in this country. It amounts to lifting the infant through the vaginal outlet, so it's less traumatic for both mother and child. Still, the use of forceps at all necessitates additional anesthesia and a larger episiotomy, which many informed women would prefer to do without.

Whether or not forceps must be used, almost all American obstetricians choose to perform an episiotomy shortly before the baby is born. This involves inserting one blade of a surgical scissors into the mother's vagina between contractions. The doctor then cuts through her perineum to enlarge the vaginal opening. Theoretically, this facilitates the birth by decreasing the pressure on the baby's head. But Mrs. H.M.I. Liley, a respected New Zealand obstetrician and author of *Modern Motherhood,* says that a slow, gradual descent through the birth canal is an important part of normal birth.

"The baby's head should not pop out," maintains Dr. Liley. If it does, the infant is "exposed in one shocking second to too much pressure change."

The typical pregnancy manual written for the general public describes an episiotomy as a relatively painless minor snipping. Most of the writers of such books, of course, are male obstetricians. Because they are men, none of them has ever experienced a "postnatal sore bottom, made all the more painful by unnecessary cutting and stitching."[29]

A few male doctors have lately become more understanding. One of them, obstetrician William J. Sweeney, explains how the double standard operates in this area. The average episiotomy is two inches long on the outside, and also two inches long on the inside. The cut extends up into the vagina, severing the muscles of the pelvic floor. Dr. Sweeney admits that a four-inch incision is traumatic in itself; the fact that a woman has to *sit* on it is outrageous. (If a *man* required a four-inch abdominal incision, it would be considered major surgery and he would be hospitalized for ten days!)

Women frequently complain about their episiotomies, not because they may be completely unnecessary, but because of the way they are repaired. Most mothers are not as unfortunate as the Canadian woman whose doctor accidentally sewed a sanitary napkin into her vagina, but many do suffer from imperfectly sutured episiotomies. Some obstetricians, in their zeal to leave their patients in perfect condition, overdo it. When the tightly sewed woman attempts to resume sexual relations, she discovers that intercourse is practically impossible; violent and persistent entry, with consequent pain to the wife, usually drives her back to the doctor to have the difficulty corrected.

Another woman found she could not reach orgasm or even enjoy sex following the birth of her fifth baby. After a time-consuming series of visits to her doctor and referrals to psychiatrists, a gynecologist discovered that a careless episiotomy repair had left her with an enlarged entrance to the vagina. Once again, corrective surgery was necessary to take care of a problem which *careless* surgery caused.

A few doctors now believe that since the perineal muscles have an eight-to-one stretch ratio, episiotomies should only be performed on those rare women who have unusually tight perineums. Yet the overwhelming majority of American doctors still perform routine episiotomies on all their maternity patients. (Except in Canada, women giving birth in other countries do not generally receive episiotomies at all.)

Doctors sometimes defend episiotomies on the grounds that they may prevent the mother's perineum from tearing if the baby's head enlarges it too suddenly. According to this theory, a straight cut is easier to suture than a jagged tear. Yet obstetricians who practice natural childbirth say that if the mother is left alone, the birth will take place with little or no damage. Furthermore, they maintain that the contractions which slowly propel the infant down the birth canal may be beneficial. They say that babies dragged out with forceps are born prematurely.

Many other people disagree with the rationale for an episiotomy because they do not think it's the baby's head that causes perineal damage. Instead, the mother's unnatural delivery position may be responsible. Spreading the mother's legs so wide constricts the pelvic outlet so that the baby needs abnormal force to navigate the birth canal. The "abducted" position that the average American mother is forced to assume during birth puts an unnatural strain upon her perineum even during normal circumstances. When the infant's head descends through the birth canal, it puts too much pressure on the woman's tightly stretched tissues.

In *Woman's Doctor*, William J. Sweeney offers another critical look at the "abducted" or dorsal lithotomy position that is almost universally used for deliveries in this country.

> . . . the woman lies on her back with her feet up in stirrups and her thighs and legs spread apart by knee rests. That puts a big strain on the perineum, and I think when we stretch the skin there so tight, we increase the chance of its tearing when the baby is born. If a lady precipitates or gives birth to a baby in bed, everything's relaxed and *usually she doesn't tear* (italics mine), or at least not as badly as when she's up in stirrups.
> . . . A woman in labor turns on her side if you leave her alone because the pain is less severe. In England, patients are delivered that way, and it's called the Sims position. But it doesn't fit in with U.S. hospital routine.[30]

English mothers who deliver in this position do not receive routine episiotomies, yet over 80 percent of them survive the birth with intact perineums or very superficial tears.[31] According to Green's *Obstetrics*, babies in New Zealand are also born with the mother lying on her side (the left lateral position). Women must lie in the dorsal lithotomy position only for operative deliveries.

In 1956, Dr. Virginia Apgar suggested that to improve the drainage of amniotic fluids, even Caesarean deliveries should be performed while the mother is lying on her side. Australian obstetricians adopted Dr. Apgar's recommendation, since she is one of the world's leading authorities on infant health. The doctors in Australia were pleased with the results of the procedure, but it has not gained acceptance in the United States.

For normal deliveries, too, the side position for birth would be measurably safer for both mother and baby. When the mother lies on her side, she prevents the weight of the unborn baby from pressing on her vena cava. (This is the large vein which collects all the blood from the legs and torso and carries it upwards to be oxygenated; it runs along the front of the spine.) If the mother lies on her back for a prolonged period of time, as she must during an American labor and delivery, the heavy uterus can squeeze the vena cava so tightly that it raises the mother's blood pressure. As the blood backs up in her inferior vena cava, circulation through the umbilical cord slows down, and the placenta swells.

This phenomenon, known as the "sluice-flow mechanism," has been a source of concern among responsible obstetricians. At a Society of Gynecologic Investigation meeting in the early 1970s, two doctors proposed a simple solution: *allow mothers to give birth on their sides* or let them use a birth stool.[32]

The ancient birth stool has reappeared in a more modern form in Sweden. Obstetrician Christman Ehrström has lately introduced an obstetrical table which is divided into two parts.

The rear half can be raised so that the mother is sitting during the delivery. This widens her pelvis and reduces the need for forceps and episiotomies. Utilizing gravity by sitting during the birth also shortens the delivery time—in some instances by many hours.[33]

Sitting was the traditional birth position in ancient Greece, ancient Rome, and throughout Europe until the nineteenth century. Sitting can further alleviate the severe back pain which the average mother must endure as the baby's head presses against the base of her spine. Sitting helps to avoid the terrible leg cramps which are frequently caused by our unnatural American delivery position. These debilitating "charley horses" can paralyze the woman's legs so badly that she can't cooperate in the delivery. Since her legs are tied to the stirrups of the delivery table, the mother's efforts to change position are doomed to frustration.

Once these leg cramps have knotted her muscles from hip to toe, the agony can reach such a crescendo that labor contractions slow down or even cease completely. This happened to me during the birth of our second baby. Since labor had gone very quickly up to that point, the doctor and several nurses were expecting the baby to be born momentarily. Yet more than twenty minutes passed without any further contractions.

"Mrs. Sousa," the doctor said, "You're not pushing hard enough!"

I tried to point to my crippled legs, but my hands were also tied down. Finally, after about twenty more minutes, the doctor injected a local anesthetic and prepared to go after the baby with forceps. Badly frightened, I began to push without stopping, and the baby was born with the help of two more contractions.

Even if the mother does not suffer excruciating leg cramps, just trying to push the baby out in this gravity-defying delivery position is an uphill task.

"From the point of view of mechanics, trying to push out

a baby with a flat back is like trying to push out a bowel movement on a bedpan while lying flat in bed."[34]

Apparently other countries do not think it necessary to put so many obstacles in the way of birth. Elisabeth Bing, cofounder of the American Society for Psychoprophylaxis in Obstetrics, estimates that fully two-thirds of the world's babies are born while the mother is squatting. There must be a reason for this, and there is. Studies have proved that squatting changes the shape of the pelvic outlet to facilitate labor. In fact, squatting is the delivery stance that is most popular in primitive countries, while lying down is *least* popular.

How can we explain the prevalence of the lying-down delivery position in our own country? Recent vibrations from the women's lib movement suggest that lying flat on the back for delivery may be far more popular with American obstetricians than it is with their patients. In *Free and Female,* Barbara Seaman asks some pointed questions about the current situation.

> Why are American women shaved, humiliated, drugged, painted and stuck up in stirrups to deliver their babies? Why are they pinned into a position which is totally unnatural and inconvenient for the mother?[35]

A passage from *Why Natural Childbirth?* echoes the same idea. Dr. Alice Rossi, a Goucher College sociologist, accuses physicians of wresting control of the childbirth experience from mothers.

> . . . I would like to put some hard questions to the medical and nursing profession. How can you strap me down like an unthinking animal on a delivery room table? How dare you claim that you "deliver" me, and cheat me of the knowledge and experience of actively giving birth to my own child. . . . The whole paraphernalia of medicine—anesthesia, strapping, the abyss below the de-

livery table—serve the function of retaining the dominant status of the attending physician.[36]

In *Husband-Coached Childbirth*, Dr. Robert Bradley makes no bones about the purposes of elaborate equipment in the delivery room.

"Such paraphernalia is designed for the convenience of the attendants only," maintains Dr. Bradley. "The mother could readily give birth in the labor room bed."

Some obstetricians have found that even raising the mother's head and shoulders on the delivery table helps to alleviate the bad effects of the dorsal lithotomy position. Comparative studies of the two positions show that propping the women resulted in shortened deliveries and less need for anesthesia. The "propped" mothers were more comfortable, more cooperative, and better able to push during the birth. Fortunately, this semisitting position is now being used more frequently in hospitals.

When women are allowed to sit up even more, equally favorable results were the rule.

"If the mother's back is elevated from the bed and flexed forward, the uterine and abdominal muscles can more naturally direct the fetus through the normal curvatures of the mother's pelvic canal, thus apparently shortening her labor," say many doctors.

While the mother is undergoing the time-consuming rigors of labor, she may not usually have anything to eat or drink. The average hospital prohibits food because of the danger of vomiting while under anesthesia. If this regulation is rigidly enforced, mothers who have long labors may become very weak and dehydrated. *Commonsense Childbirth* tells how Mrs. Hazell, the author, went without food or water for thirty-eight hours during her first delivery.

For the past twenty-five years or so, nutritionists have been trying to teach how important food is during times of stress, such as illness or labor. Adelle Davis recommended eating a hearty, protein-rich snack at the beginning of labor. To maintain strength during labor, she advised the mother to sip Pep-up (a fortified blended milk drink) every few hours. Some nutritionists realize that woman's need for every vitamin and nutrient increases drastically during labor. According to *Let's Have Healthy Children,* the right foods, plenty of water, and even vitamin and mineral supplements can shorten labor, ease delivery, and lessen maternal bleeding.

A manual for rural midwives also stresses the vital role of nutrition during labor. It advises them to give food at regular intervals, and to offer water to the mother in labor every hour. Since they have little medical equipment to fall back on, these young midwives have to rely on natural means to maintain their patient's strength and to help her not become exhausted during labor.

When the American mother is almost ready to deliver, she is moved from her labor room bed to a high, narrow table in the delivery room. Once she is strapped into position, a nurse may show her how to grasp the iron handgrips. Often, she is told to push as if she were trying to move her bowels.

But if the woman actually strains like this, she contracts her rectal muscles and compresses the vaginal opening. (By a reflex contraction, bearing down against the rectum hardens the perineum.) Mobilizing and tightening the muscles of the pelvic floor thus creates another obstacle for the baby's head. To overcome this barrier, the uterus and abdominal muscles have to work twice as hard—lengthening the delivery and increasing the pain. In *Thank You, Dr. Lamaze,* a book about the early days of natural childbirth, the author was warned by her French midwife that pushing with a tight perineum could actually *double* her delivery time!

Some experts think that the mother should not push until the very end of labor, as the baby's head is actually being born. Before this final stage, they claim, straining will only cause pain to the mother, and decrease the supply of blood and oxygen to the baby. Even during the final moments, no more pushing is usually necessary than that which the body does irresistibly, as in defecation.[37]

I followed this advice when our last two babies were born at home, and it worked beautifully. It seems much more sensible to push only when one's body demands it. Our fourth baby was born very fast and I didn't have to bear down at all. With our fifth baby, though, I did. She was born after a weak, irregular labor, and needed a bit of extra help to emerge. During her birth, I pushed only twice: once to deliver her head and once to deliver her shoulders.

Anyone who has delivered a baby in an American hospital will appreciate how revolutionary this idea is. It's helpful to realize that whether or not the mother does any pushing at all, her uterus is perfectly capable of doing the job all by itself. The strongest muscle in the human body, the female uterus exerts about fifty pounds of force during a contraction. "Women can go through labor heavily sedated, unconscious, or in a coma."[38]

Unfortunately, the average American delivery room is a very noisy, tense place. Whenever the laboring mother has a contraction, the nurses and doctor loudly command her to push, push, and keep on pushing. Their shouts may be punctuated by the woman's screams of protest. This could be the reason why.

> If the woman is pushing hard because she feels this is what is expected of her in the second stage and not because her uterine conditions demand it, or because she senses an atmosphere of haste or urgency, or if she is pushing against an as yet inadequately dilated perineum, the feeling she experiences will be one of extreme discomfort.[39]

With the mother tied down hand and foot, and possibly having her face covered with a mask, it's only natural that she might think that following orders to push is her only alternative. But such premature straining can be not only painful, but dangerous. A study found that when mothers were allowed to push only when they felt the desire to bear down, their deliveries were much less complicated than the deliveries of women who were forced to follow orders to push from their birth attendants. The mothers who were given the freedom to decide when they wanted to bear down needed fewer episiotomies and less anesthesia. Also, forceps were needed in far fewer cases.

A common practice in U.S. delivery rooms is for the mother to receive a hormone shot as the baby is being born. This stimulates the uterus to contract and decreases the possibility of hemorrhaging. Sometimes, however, the uterus contracts so violently that the placenta is retained. When this happens, the doctor must remove it by hand. Usually he has to reach up into the uterus, detach the placenta, and scoop or scrape it out. In recent years this procedure has been questioned by many who are concerned about maternal health. The author of *Commonsense Childbirth* condemns it; she believes that tearing out the placenta increases the chances of starting uterine or vaginal infections.

Some obstetricians also think that when the doctor reaches his hand up into the mother's uterus, he may introduce a bit of the infant's blood into her bloodstream. If there is a possibility of Rh incompatibility, the mother should be carefully guarded against this. Just one drop of the baby's blood can cause her body to start manufacturing antibodies against it, thus jeopardizing any future children she might bear.

According to Green's *Obstetrics,* "manipulation of the fundus and an excessive number of attempts at expressing the placenta before it is separated are potent causes of maternal shock." Suddenly tearing the placenta off the uterine wall, instead of letting it detach itself gradually, can result in heavy bleeding. Hemorrhage, one of the leading causes of maternal death in the United States, is chiefly associated with excessive intrauterine manipulation and the questionable use of oxytocic drugs which cause the uterus to rupture, according to the 1968 Report on Confidential Inquiries into Maternal Deaths in the District of Columbia. Citing physician negligence and too much obstetrical interference with normal births, the author of this publication estimated that about half of our yearly maternal fatalities could be prevented.

Thanks to easily available blood transfusions, the average American mother is not likely to die during delivery. She has no similar protection, however, against the emotional and psychic damage our traditional birth customs may cause, as the following example shows.

One young lady, eager to have her baby as naturally as possible, finally located an obstetrician who agreed to "allow" natural childbirth provided she would "take his advice on anesthetics if *he* felt the situation called for it." Three hours after arriving at the hospital, she received a cervical block and Pitocin to stimulate her labor. When she protested and became panicky, the attendants gave her a hypo and then full anesthesia. The obstetrician had to deliver her baby with forceps, and she hemorrhaged after the birth. Blood transfusions were given, and the mother finally woke up lying in the intensive care unit, groggy with Nembutal. When the nurse finally brought her baby girl, she was "beyond even feigning joy."

After going through an experience like this, is it any wonder that so many American mothers suffer from postpartum depression? This syndrome is now so common in the country that it has become an expected and accepted part of our American way of birth. Since the effects of postpartum depression can be serious and long-lasting, some childbirth authorities have called for a comprehensive investigation of its causes. Our routine methods of delivery may play an important part in creating postpartum depression. Besides the rigors of labor and delivery, the many extra stresses imposed by the hospital often contribute to feelings of helplessness and confusion in new mothers. Many women also feel guilty about their loss of control under the influence of childbirth drugs.

Mothers who have received scopolamine or anesthesia often experience feelings of unease and unreality about the "missing days" of their lives.[40]

Recent studies at Stanford University suggest that postpartum depression is most likely to be felt by mothers who have difficult labors, by mothers who are having their first babies, and by mothers who suffer significant postdelivery discomfort. In *Methods of Childbirth,* Constance Bean notes that "the prepared childbirth experience with the emotional support which it provides is a great help in preventing or reducing these feelings which are so common in the traditional childbirth experience."[41] Unfortunately, prepared childbirth is still only available to a small minority of American mothers.

Lately, more suspicion has focused upon the hospital itself as a primary cause of postpartum blues.

"From my observation, this depression is far less experienced in a home birth situation than is commonly reported to exist in hospitals," states a California midwife. Physicians who are active in the home delivery field confirm this opinion.

Alternative birth methods, such as prepared or family-centered childbirth, require psychological support from the obstetrician. In spite of the proven success of these techniques in countries like France and the Soviet Union, most American doctors do not seem to be willing to exert their energies in these directions. Instead, they tend to rely ever more heavily upon the technical aspects of obstetrical care. During the past five years, many new hospital procedures have come into increasing use on our maternity wards. An example of these is the routine administration of intravenous feedings of glucose or dextrose and water to all maternity patients.

Obstetricians offer various reasons for this annoying practice. Some say it may help the woman to avoid becoming weak and dehydrated, since she is not allowed to drink water. (In 1974, however, a Harvard Medical School surgeon discovered that the standard intravenous dextrose solution dissipated the body's essential proteins more quickly than if the patients received nothing at all!)

Other obstetricians like to have an I.V. in place so they can administer Pitocin intravenously. Most doctors agree, though, that one of the most important reasons for inserting an I.V. is that if the woman has a sudden hemorrhage, it would be easier to give her a transfusion.

I questioned a hospital chief of obstetrics about the percentage of mothers who did, in fact, require postpartum transfusions. He estimated that well under one percent of their patients needed such emergency care.

"Then why," I wondered, "do you make the other 99 percent get an I.V. anyway?"

Is it fair to subject a normal, healthy woman to an unnecessary, sometimes painful, and always cumbersome I.V.? What about the risks of hepatitis, swelling, infections, and other complications which may be associated with intravenous equipment? While most side effects of I.V.s are relatively minor, some are not. In 1974, a Sacramento, California girl received a contaminated intravenous solution which caused her to go blind, according to a suit filed in California Superior Court.

"The routine use of intravenous fluids, without special reason, is annoying and unnecessary," states *Methods of Childbirth*. I agree completely. In fact, this was one of the reasons why I had my last two babies at home. In the early 1970s, Air Force hospitals began insisting that all their maternity patients have routine intravenous glucose solutions. My record of previous normal births made no difference; if I wanted to have a baby at a military hospital, I would have to accept an I.V.

Hooked up to an I.V. bottle, a mother who is in labor cannot get up and go to the bathroom. Experts recommend that she should empty her bladder every two hours, but an I.V. makes this impossible. If her labor is a long one, she might have to be catheterized. Inserting a rubber catheter into the bladder to drain off the urine is one of the leading causes of urinary disease, according to obstetrician William Sweeney.

"There are more infections and problems caused by inserting a tube through that dirty urethra from below than you would believe," declares Dr. Sweeney.

Unfortunately, by the time the woman in labor needs to be catheterized, it is far too late for her to discuss the risks of urinary infections with her doctor.

Researchers have noted that many young couples are being so "turned off" by the threat of this type of hospital procedure that they choose to have their babies at home.

"They should know that they do have the right to refuse these procedures if they wish," says Constance A. Bean.

The true state of affairs is usually far from being that simple. Many hospitals give the patient no choice about what is done to her. Military hospitals, for example, offer their care on a "take it or leave it" basis. If a military dependent refuses to accept part of the standard maternity care "menu," the hospital will not give her the medical care she is entitled to by law. Thus a military wife who refuses an I.V. must have her baby in a civilian hospital. (Some women have been successful in forcing hospitals to treat them without accepting infusions and transfusions, but they have occasionally had to take the hospital to court.)

Municipal hospitals which accept a high proportion of welfare patients are said to be even more authoritarian in these matters. *Our Bodies, Ourselves* contains many examples of how "the poor take more." In general, the less the patient personally pays for her care, the less control she has over any aspect of her treatment. It's obvious that large groups of women, including welfare recipients, military dependents, unmarried mothers and the mentally disabled have little, if any, control over their birth experiences.

"When the pregnant woman is young and unmarried, the doctor's contempt is only slightly greater than that exhibited toward a menopausal woman who accidentally conceives," reports *Vaginal Politics.*

"At City Hospital, where the patient load is heavily nonwhite and poor, the worst treatment was observed," according to *Forced Labor.* [42] In addition, this study found that City Hospital staff addressed maternity patients by number, rather than by name, limited their visiting hours, didn't try to teach the mothers postpartum hygiene, and allowed them to feed their babies for a *total* of only two hours a day, instead of the usual five or six hours!

Occasionally, poor or uninformed mothers have been permanently sterilized without their knowledge following childbirth. In a 1974 claim, three California women sought damages from Los Angeles County, arguing that they gave permission for their sterilizations while they were in pain during labor, and under heavy sedation. Fortunately, such mishaps have been relatively rare.

Another recent technological development that may be inflicted upon a laboring mother is the fetal monitor. This device, which measures the baby's heartbeat while it is still in the womb, can be a boon in certain high-risk deliveries. As of 1972, however, there existed "no evidence that it adds safety and is the change needed to improve the infant death rate."[43] Then the question arises as to whether such a sophisticated piece of equipment ought to be used routinely for normal deliveries. If it is, then parents who want natural childbirth may be made to feel negligent if they do not want to use the monitor.

One of the fetal monitoring devices calls for a plate to be strapped to the mother's leg. From this plate run wires in two directions—one to the mother and one to the baby. One of the electrodes must be placed in the mother's uterus via her vagina. *Methods of Childbirth* warns that "there may be some discomfort from this procedure."

"More births in the near tomorrow will take place in a setting of blinking lights, green glowing cathode-ray screens, dials and wires and tubes. For patients who do not know what to expect, the effect at first may be frightening," according to *New Miracles of Childbirth.* So besides producing pain, the fetal monitor may also produce fright.

If the insertion of the monitor's electrodes can cause fear

and pain in the mother, what about its effect on her baby? One of the wires must be hooked up to the infant's scalp. The pinpricks caused by the insertion of the electrodes will be visible on the baby's head for several days after his birth. Despite the well-known fact that the unborn infant can feel pain, there has been little concern about the possible trauma to him from the use of fetal monitors. Subjecting a normal infant to unnecessary pain simply because the advanced stage of our technology makes it possible seems terribly heartless.

Being "wired for sound" is only one of the hazards that face the average baby born in an American hospital today. The following chapter explains some of the other risks he may encounter.

NOTES

1. Natalie Gittelson, "Midwives?" *Harper's Bazaar*, June 1972, p. 105.
2. Deborah Tanzer and Jean L. Block, *Why Natural Childbirth?* (Garden City, New York: Doubleday & Co., 1972), pp. 145-149.
3. Aljean Harmetz, "The Way Childbirth *Really* Is," *Today's Health*, February 1972, p. 30.
4. The Boston Children's Medical Center, *Pregnancy, Birth and the Newborn Baby* (Boston: Boston Children's Medical Center, 1971), p. 52.
5. Lester Dessez Hazell, *Commonsense Childbirth* (New York: G.P. Putnam's Sons, 1969), p. 11.
6. Sheldon H. Cherry, M.D., *Understanding Pregnancy and Childbirth* (Indianapolis: Bobbs-Merrill, 1973), p. 80.
7. Elisabeth Bing, *The Adventure of Birth* (New York: Simon & Schuster, 1970), p. 116.
8. Aljean Harmetz, op. cit., p. 32.
9. Constance A. Bean, *Methods of Childbirth* (Garden City, N.Y.: Doubleday & Co., 1972), p. 28.
10. Sheldon H. Cherry, op. cit., p. 80.
11. Nancy Stoller Shaw, *Forced Labor: Maternity Care in the United States,* (Elmsford, N.Y.: Pergamon Press, 1974), p. 76.
12. Ibid.
13. Elliott H. McCleary, *New Miracles of Childbirth* (New York: David McKay, 1974), p. 104.

14. *National Right To Life News,* "Vital Signs," (Nine to Five Obstetrics?), February 1975, p. 10.
15. Suzanne Arms, "How Hospitals Complicate Childbirth," *Ms.,* May 1975, p. 108.
16. Ibid., p. 109.
17. Lester D. Hazell, op. cit., p. 138.
18. Irwin Chabon, M.D., *Awake and Aware,* (New York: Delacorte Press, 1966), p. 66.
19. Sheldon H. Cherry, op. cit., p. 81.
20. Elliott H. McCleary, op. cit., p. 38.
21. The Boston Women's Health Book Collective, *Our Bodies, Ourselves* (New York: Simon & Schuster, 1971), p. 248.
22. Constance A. Bean, op. cit., p. 129.
23. Wayne L. Johnson, "Regionals Can Prolong Labor," *Medical World News,* October 15, 1971, p. 41 (cited in *Our Bodies, Ourselves,* p. 195).
24. Arthur Gorbach, M.D., "What to Expect During Labor and Delivery," *Redbook,* December 1972, p. 67.
25. Barbara Seaman, *Free and Female* (New York: Coward, McCann & Geoghegan, 1972), p. 155.
26. Constance A. Bean, op. cit., p. 192.
27. Elliott H. McCleary, op. cit., pp. 201-202.
28. Sheldon H. Cherry, op. cit., p. 83.
29. Shirley Streshinsky, "Are You Safer With a Midwife?" *Ms.,* October 1973, p. 24.
30. William J. Sweeney III, M.D. with Barbara Lang Stern, *Woman's Doctor,* (New York: Wm. Morrow & Co., 1973), pp. 273-275.
31. Niles Newton, *Maternal Emotions* (New York: Paul E. Hoeber, Inc., 1955), p. 39.
32. Barbara Seaman, op. cit., p. 143.
33. "Sit Down, Have a Baby," *Newsweek,* May 21, 1973, p. 72.
34. The Boston Children's Medical Center, op. cit., p. 26.
35. Seaman, op. cit., p. 142.
36. Tanzer, op. cit., p. 251.
37. H.M.I. Liley, M.D., and Beth Day, *Modern Motherhood* (New York: Random House, 1969), p. 66.
38. Ibid., p. 78.
39. Sheila Kitzinger, *The Experience of Childbirth* (New York: Taplinger Publishing Company, 1962), p. 202.
40. The Boston Children's Medical Center, op. cit., p. 193.
41. Constance A. Bean, op. cit., p. 137.
42. Shaw, op. cit., p. 123.
43. Bean, op. cit., p. 166.

OTHER SOURCES
(listed as they appear in text)

Germaine Greer, *The Female Eunuch* (New York: McGraw-Hill Book Co. 1970), p. 39.

Donald Robinson, "The Newest Major Advances in Hospital Care," *Parade*, October 27, 1974, p. 7.

Alan F. Guttmacher, M.D., *Pregnancy, Birth and Family Planning* (New York: The Viking Press, 1973), p. 192.

F.E. Shideman, M.D., *Take As Directed* (Minneapolis: Chemical Rubber Company, 1967), p. 147.

Derek Llewellyn-Jones, M.D., *Everywoman and Her Body* (New York: Taplinger Publishing Company, 1971), p. 244.

Virginia Apgar and Joan Beck, *Is My Baby All Right?* (New York: Trident Press, 1972).

"Malpractice Settlement May Top $1.2 Million," *The Sacramento Union*, Sacramento, California, December 4, 1973, A3.

Michelle Landsberg, "Your Gynecologist," *Chatelaine*, August 1973, p. 65.

George Herbert Green, M.D., *Introduction to Obstetrics* (Christchurch: E.M. Peryer Ltd., 1966.)

Robert A. Bradley, M.D., *Husband-Coached Childbirth* (New York: Harper & Row, 1965), p. 17.

Helen Wessel, *Natural Childbirth and the Family* (New York: Harper & Row, 1973.)

Adelle Davis, *Let's Have Healthy Children* (New York: Harcourt Brace Jovanovich, 1973), p. 153.

Instituto Indigenista Interamericano, *Pregnancy, Childbirth and the Newborn* (Mexico City, 1959), p. 60.

Marjorie Karmel, *Thank You, Dr. Lamaze* (Philadelphia: J.B. Lippincott Company, 1959), p. 60.

"Do Americans Starve? Yes, in Hospitals," *The Sacramento Bee*, Sacramento, California, March 29, 1974, p. A 21.

"Parents File Malpractice Suit," *The Sacramento Bee*, Sacramento, California, April 5, 1974, p. B 1.

"Court Affirms Woman's Right to Pick Death," *The Sacramento Bee*, April 26, 1974, p. A 20.

Ellen Frankfort, *Vaginal Politics* (New York: Quadrangle Books, 1972), p. 38.

"L.A. Women File Suit in Sterilization Case," *The Sacramento Bee*, Sacramento, California, November 21, 1974, p. A 14.

3

WHAT ABOUT THE BABY?

While ample consideration has been given to the mother during labor and delivery, the baby's experience has received but scant attention until recently. Research at the Menninger Foundation in Topeka suggests that the unborn infant is much further developed than was previously suspected. While still in the womb, the baby learns to suck its thumb and swallow.[1] By the time it's born, the baby may be drinking a quart of amniotic fluid daily. Loud noises make the unborn infant jump; he dodges to avoid pain. We still have much to learn about fetal development, but one thing is clear: the unborn baby is not insensitive.

When the time for birth is at hand, the uterus periodically hardens and squeezes its contents "against the tightly closed neck of the womb, the cervix, opening it little by little."[2] As long as the mother's pelvic floor remains perfectly relaxed, these uterine contractions alone can produce delivery in a rhythmic, coordinated manner. Like digestion, birth is a normal physiological process that works best if left alone. The uterus, unaided, will not only propel the baby through the birth canal, but will also regulate his descent so he can gradually get used to the change in pressure. (Of course, when forceps are used to pull the infant out, these natural birth mechanisms are circumvented.)

If the baby is allowed to be born spontaneously, he usually cries as soon as his head emerges, or within a few seconds after he is born. Good color, vigorous kicking and arm waving, and steady breathing should be the norm during the baby's first few minutes of life. In these respects, observers have found infants born to unmedicated mothers so far superior to conventional-childbirth babies that they have begun to question our entire standard of neonatal behavior. Argentinian doctors who have made similar comparisons discovered that the reflex function of newborn natural-childbirth infants equals the reflexes of four-day-old infants who were delivered conventionally.[3]

If a woman has been medicated or anesthetized during labor, her baby is far more apt to look blue, to be limp, and not to breathe unless resuscitative methods are used. This is not too surprising. The first few breaths of air will be difficult for *any* baby, as he must inflate thousands of previously unused air sacs in his lungs. It's estimated that the newborn baby requires at least five times the effort that we do to fill his lungs with air during the first moments of life.[4] If the infant's respiratory center is depressed, however, he will hardly be able to make this effort without help.

In spite of resuscitative efforts, many of these babies don't survive. *Natural Childbirth and the Family* points out that approximately 60 percent of neonatal deaths in our country occur because of lack of oxygen, "partly because of improper use of drugs." For this reason, Dr. Ralph Gause, obstetrics chief of New York's Roosevelt Hospital, urged doctors to withhold the traditionally administered sedatives and anesthetics from mothers. He estimated that in 1968, there were "about five million partially damaged children in this country, many of which were due to minor injuries during labor and delivery."

Most experts in this area admit that whatever medication is given to the mother during labor, there is always some danger to her child. Yet "it is known that in normal instances birth will be effected without detriment to mother or child if no drugs are given to the mother." Because of this, increasing numbers of conscientious physicians recommend that all childbirth drugs should be used only by exception—that is, when there is a clear-cut need for their help.

A few years ago, pediatrician T. Berry Brazelton investigated the results of depressant childbirth drugs on the newborn infant. Dr. Brazelton discovered that because of the immaturity of the newborn's kidneys, it can take over a week for his system to detoxify these substances. In the meantime, the baby acts sleepy, listless, unresponsive, and sometimes disoriented. Typically, he may suffer frequent breathing crises; when he chokes and turns blue, nurses must help him to recover in time.

Sadly, these effects are usually not explained to the infant's mother. If she has not been told why her baby is temporarily unable to respond like a normal infant, she will probably wonder what's wrong with him. She may even suspect that the baby has a serious illness which the doctors are hiding from her. If she tries to nurse the baby, her suspicions may be confirmed by the way he lacks interest. When the drugged baby refuses to nurse, the emotional turmoil created in the mother's mind acts to further decrease her milk supply.

These conditions have been confirmed by many studies. When mothers received barbiturates and anesthetics during labor, their babies had difficulties in nursing and did not gain weight for several days. Babies born to unmedicated mothers, however, were nursing well and gaining weight by the third day of their lives.[5]

Another research team at the University of Pennsylvania recently discovered that when mothers receive barbiturate sedation during labor, their babies show disturbances in their sucking ability. A machine, similar to that which records

brain-wave activity, can measure and graph the infant's sucking pattern. When mothers receive barbiturates, their babies'
sucking is slower and less consistent than normal. This
machine was once used to measure the sucking patterns of a
pair of twins. The first twin, who had been born naturally,
showed rhythmic, efficient sucking behavior; the other twin,
who had been delivered by forceps, showed abnormal sucking
rhythms for six weeks.[6] (As his sucking pattern became normal, doctors were able to tell the mother that he had not
suffered permanent brain damage.)

Routine use of obstetrical medication is the main difference between American birth customs and those in countries
which have better infant mortality rates, such as Holland,
Sweden, England, and Japan. Although many doctors are
wont to place the blame for our high infant death rate upon
lack of prenatal care, premature births, and other factors out
of their control, these conditions also exist in other countries
with better birth records.

"Deprivation, birth defects, prematurity and low birth
weight are not unique to the United States, and 40 percent to
60 percent of early infant deaths occur in full-term infants of
birth weight over five and a half pounds," according to
Methods of Childbirth. Therefore we have no choice but to look
to our particular obstetrical peculiarities to find out why more
newborns die in America than in over a dozen other compa-
rable countries.

When questioned about our high neonatal mortality rate,
many doctors attribute it to the non-white births in the United
States. According to their theory, the death rate of babies born
to black, Hispanic and Indian mothers is greater than white
infants, which tends to lower the national figures. But a 1970
Carnegie Commission study deflated this theory after it investigated the neonatal death rates of *white* babies *only.* According
to their report, our white infants died at the rate of almost
twenty per 1,000, which is still higher than ten of the countries
that outrank us.[7]

Besides running a greater danger of not surviving his own birth, the average American infant also faces high risks in other areas. Neurological defects, cerebral palsy, spinal and brain injuries, and behavior disorders are only a few of the conditions which may be caused by birth-connected trauma. A shocking one out of every sixteen American babies suffers from birth defects!

Out of every thirty-three babies born today, one will be a victim of either mental retardation or cerebral palsy. As long ago as the 1940s, physicians concerned about this country's extremely high rate of cerebral palsy identified the following factors as being probably responsible:

1. Lack of oxygen before and after birth, caused by the injudicious use of obstetric analgesia and anesthesia

2. Prolonged labor and traumatic delivery

3. Brain traumata caused by improper application of forceps

Yet our delivery customs hang on, and so does our unbelievably high incidence of cerebral palsy—almost 500 per 100,000 births, according to the United Cerebral Palsy Foundation. With approximately 15,000 new cases of cerebral palsy each year in the United States, we maintain an unenviable record. "Our country has a greater percentage of cerebral-palsied children in proportion to our population than any other nation in the world."[8]

A significant percentage of children born with cerebral palsy have normal or above-average intelligence. But because of their handicap, it is very difficult for them to learn from their environment. Later on, the spastic youngster may be placed in special classes or schools, where he gradually falls behind his contemporaries. The rare child who is able to buck the system and graduate from school may then find himself unable to find work.

A young writer in Sacramento, California is now in this predicament. Although he is a college graduate, his cerebral palsy prevents him from being employed, so he does part-time volunteer work with handicapped children. In spite of his outgoing personality, social life is almost impossible; his constant drooling makes both eating and talking very difficult. It's easy to understand why one therapist describes growing up with cerebral palsy as a "long series of emotional shocks."

Recently, additional abnormalities have been traced to medicated childbirth. Lower intelligence, short attention spans, deafness, behavior problems, and learning difficulties are just a few of the effects which experts think may result from over-use of modern delivery drugs. Many other parents can recount experiences like this story related by Mrs. Marjie Hathaway.

> Our twelve-year-old son is having some reading problems. We've been told by doctors that it is because of the medication I was given during his birth. What gripes me is that I never asked for any medication. They just give it. You have no choice. You are just a lowly woman. They say, "We will give you all this medication and don't you worry about a thing!" Nobody says to you, "Hey, that might harm your baby. That might mean that when he's twelve years old, he will have problems."[9]

Another set of parents did not get off as easily as the Hathaways. A jury awarded them half a million dollars in 1968 to care for their birth-damaged child. It was charged that their baby's gross mental retardation resulted primarily from an injection of Demerol which was given to his mother shortly before a premature delivery.

Demerol is one of the most popular obstetrical analgesics, but when it is given too close to the baby's birth, it inhibits the infant's respiratory center. In *The Gist of Obstetrics,* Dr. H.B. Atlee claims that up to 67 percent of babies whose mothers receive such depressants fail to breathe spontaneously. Compare this to the performance of infants born to unmedicated mothers. Only 2 percent of them need help to start breathing.

It is obvious that doubts are arising on all sides about the wisdom of bringing babies into the world with their tiny bodies clogged with potentially harmful drugs. It has been suggested, and not in jest, that one explanation for the Soviets' head start in outer space may be found in their nonmedication of mothers at birth, thereby producing babies whose brains function better.[10]

If a newborn baby does not breathe spontaneously, he must be helped with various suction tubes and oxygenating devices; cool water and slapping his feet also may be tried. But most experts now agree that even a short delay in breathing may have a definite connection with mental retardation, cerebral palsy, learning disabilities, and neurological abnormalities. According to a 1973 book, "The longer it takes to start him breathing adequately, the more likely that the baby who survives will have brain damage and the greater this damage will be."

Besides causing lethargy and breathing difficulties in newborn infants, some doctors fear that giving the mother drugs may be responsible for the increasing incidence of amniotic fluid contamination. When the baby's oxygen supply is decreased, because delivery drugs lower the mother's blood pressure, the infant's efforts to obtain oxygen often cause him to expel meconium while still in the womb. If the baby later inhales the contaminated amniotic fluid, serious lung problems may develop during his first week of life.

Another potential source of danger to the unborn baby is the use of Pitocin or other oxytocic hormones to induce or hasten labor. Not only do these drugs occasionally rupture the mother's uterus, they can also increase both the length and strength of her contractions so much that the baby's oxygen supply runs short. In fact one recent study discovered that almost three out of every four such oxytocin-induced contractions decreased the amount of oxygen reaching the infant's brain! These figures were obtained from fetal monitor tracings.

Pitocin and oxytocin, unless administered with utmost caution, can also cause a precipitate delivery. When this happens, the strong uterine contractions get out of control and eject the baby too quickly. The sudden change from the intrauterine environment may result in bleeding in the infant's brain.[11]

Once the baby is born, state law usually requires that prophylactic medication be placed in his eyes. This is to prevent blindness, if the baby's eyes have contacted the gonococcus germ. A mother who has gonorrhea can transmit the bacteria as the baby passes through her birth canal, but a weak silver nitrate solution will kill any germs the baby might have picked up. If the silver nitrate solution is too strong, however, it can permanently blind the infant. Unfortunately, such accidents have occurred several times in the past.

Even in its correct dilution, silver nitrate "may cause considerable swelling around the eyes, sometimes enough to hide them entirely, and also a temporary discharge."[12] Many hospitals now use antibiotic ointments in place of silver nitrate, but they are not always effective. Parents often question whether their baby has to receive even this medication. If the mother has never been exposed to gonorrhea, why must her baby be subjected to such treatment at all? Rather than inflame every baby's eyes with medication, some doctors suggest testing the mother for gonorrhea shortly before she delivers. Antibiotics could then be given to *her,* or to *her baby,* instead of imposed on all babies.

Although most of the hospital care given to newborns is good, an occasional oversight can result in needless tragedy. Here is an example of how our haphazard system of maternity care claims innocent victims.

On a chilly January afternoon, the temperature of the delivery room was so cold that the nurses were wearing sweaters and coats. After a normal birth, the doctor told the mother that her baby looked and sounded perfect. Since it had been a natural childbirth, the mother was awake.

The doctor put the newborn baby on a nearby table while

he attended to the mother's episiotomy repair. Naked and crying, the infant slowly turned from pink to blue, as the helpless mother watched, horrified. After about five minutes, the baby's cries suddenly stopped, and a nurse alerted the doctor.

Although an airlock incubator was at hand for such emergencies, the doctor gave oxygen to the baby via a "relatively primitive method." Consequently, the infant's struggles caused most of the oxygen to escape from the funnel. After about forty-five minutes of this, the doctor sent the baby to the nursery, never checked on her again, and left no special orders for her care.

Three days later, the infant's condition had deteriorated so badly that she was placed on the critical list. By then, the exposure, shock and oxygen deprivation had caused irreversible brain damage. This baby, who was born "perfect," is now a small girl. She is blind and deaf. She can't feel or talk. She cannot control her muscles, and she has periodic convulsions.

The hospital environment often seems almost designed to neglect many of the infant's basic needs. For example, simple instinct tells most of the world's mothers that the baby probably feels insecure and chilly during his first few moments of extrauterine life. Since the baby has spent nine months in a small space and a warm temperature of 98.6°, we can easily appreciate how hostile our world must seem to him. A mother's natural response to her baby's first screams is to wrap him up warmly and hold him securely. Almost unconsciously, mothers try to comfort their newborn infants by cradling them in their arms, holding them on the left side. This response is so universal that anthropologists call it the baby-rocking position, noting that little girls usually hold their dolls like this, too.

Since the mother's heart is on her left side, it would be logical to conclude that instinct prompts her to hold her baby where he can hear a sound that has been familiar to him during his prenatal days. In fact, when a tape recording of mothers' heartbeats was played in a nursery of newborn babies, they digested their food better, grew faster, and were happier than babies who did not hear the heartbeats.

In another experiment to learn more about the newborn's earliest needs, Dr. Harry Harlow separated rhesus monkeys from their mothers soon after birth. When the baby monkeys were later offered a variety of mechanical mother substitutes, they consistently chose the dummies that were soft and warm. Even if the surrogate "mother" looked nothing like a real monkey, the orphaned rhesus infants always thought that softness and warmth were more important than appearance.

How do hospitals meet these needs of the newborn baby? Certainly not by leaving him naked while he is weighed, measured, cleaned and medicated. The typical American infant must also suffer such routine procedures as forceps delivery, fetal monitoring devices, vitamin K injections, and irritating eyedrops. While the baby is still screaming from all these annoyances, he is often unceremoniously deposited in the nursery to hear other babies crying. According to one authority, however, the baby "needs the physical contact of being held before being wheeled down to be added to the row of cribs in the nursery. Gentle handling helps to stimulate his breathing and circulation."[13]

Recent studies prove that the newborn infant is much more advanced than was thought before. He can hear very well, he can see, and he can even respond to what he sees. A Menninger Foundation researcher, Dr. Joseph Kovach, says that a baby can smile during the first ten minutes of its life. If the mother smiles back at him, he receives the stimulus to smile again, thus starting a private communication system.

It's now believed that these early interactions are extremely important, since they may form the foundations of language. If the mother is not there to return the baby's smile, or if some other part of the interaction is missing, psychological disorders may be in store for the infant later in life.

When the mother has to lie in a recovery room for several hours, she can't experience the thrill of getting acquainted with her new baby. Hospital rules, which were made when mothers needed to recover from heavy anesthesia, sometimes prohibit the mother from having her baby for up to an entire day. When the mother is not allowed to see her baby for hours, she may feel very anxious about his safety, especially if her memory of the birth is foggy from delivery drugs.

If the mother asks for her baby, the nurses may try to reassure her. They may tell her that the baby needs constant observation during the first day. To the mother, it sounds as if he can receive good care only in the specialized surroundings of the nursery. But how true is this?

> It is a myth for anyone, doctor or parent, to assume that each baby in the nursery is actually watched constantly, that his needs for holding and feeding are met in the nursery, and that his care is a medical responsibility which no ordinary mortal could assume. The care system has not been set up that way to provide individual care continually. The use of monitoring equipment would not be the answer for providing constant observation either, but would simply offer another way of dehumanizing the care of the new baby.[14]

Frequently, American doctors justify the need for centralized baby care by saying that the nursery protects the newborn from germs; yet obstetricians in other countries do not believe that this is necessarily the best thing for him. Dr. H.M.I. Liley, a prominent New Zealand obstetrician, explains why.

"It is artificial and unnecessary to 'protect' the newborn from bacteria (unless he is premature) by isolating him in an antiseptic nursery, away from his mother's bacteria and emotions. The newborn must get harmless bacteria all over his skin surface as soon as possible if he is to survive this germ-filled world."

Just how efficiently does the hospital nursery protect newborn babies from germs, anyway? In many instances, instead of being protected from harmful bacteria, newborn infants are exposed to them.

Hospital-bred staph infections can cause infant diarrhea, boils, impetigo, and even pneumonia. One particularly contagious germ is sometimes picked up by the baby in the hospital and transmitted to its mother when she nurses the baby. The mother who develops painful breast abscesses may not connect them with her hospital stay, until her doctor enlightens her when she returns to him for treatment.

Another factor which makes these infections even more obnoxious is the fact that hospital-bred germs are resistant to many antiobiotics. Thus, the mother or baby unfortunate enough to catch one may be in for a long and annoying and expensive battle against the hardy microbe. Also, when hospital nurseries stopped using the antibacterial hexachlorophene, "hospital-acquired infections rose dramatically to new heights."[15]

One American university hospital puts the babies' cribs next to their mothers' beds during the day, returning them to a central nursery at 9 P.M. Despite the increased exposure of the infants to other adults—(four mothers occupy each room)—there has been no rate increase in infection. Women who have this "modified" rooming-in plan react favorably not only to the arrangement, but toward their entire hospital experience. They welcome the opportunity to have their own babies and to learn from the other mothers in the room. Because of their resulting high morale, nurses find it easier to care for these patients. Much of the infant care is reduced, too, because each woman can respond to the immediate needs of her own baby.[16]

Besides the baby's basic physical needs, he also has psychological and emotional necessities. His need to be close to his mother is recognized in most cultures, and studies of animals tend to emphasize how basic such behavior can be.

When newborn goats or lambs are removed from their mothers immediately after birth, observers note a decrease of maternal responsiveness to the baby's needs, a weaker attachment between mother and baby, and sometimes even rejection or mild attack by the mother. The infant animals respond to early separation by developing split-personality symptoms. When they mature, they often are unable to mate with the opposite sex. If they do become parents, they don't know how to take care of their own babies very well.

In spite of such experimental evidence, American birth procedures remove the baby from his mother almost immediately. We treat our children as independent entities as soon as the umbilical cord has been cut. Separating the baby from his mother so early may be responsible for the fretfulness and overdependence of so many young American children, according to anthropologist Margaret Mead. Without a doubt, American mothers seem to rely more on infant seats, playpens and walker-chairs than mothers in other countries. It would be interesting to find out to what extent our customs of childbirth are responsible for our particular styles of baby care.

Many experts feel that the rigid schedule of a hospital nursery "does not have the proper regard for the newborn baby's needs nor for the particular stresses of the mother in her adjustment to her new environment."[17] Dr. Edith B. Jackson, former Yale professor of Pediatric Psychiatry, summarized the newborn's basic requirements as follows:

> The first [infantile] needs of the child according to present tenets, are prompt satisfaction of hunger and of the urge to nuzzle and suck, a feeling of warmth and support from a nurturing mother, and a peaceful undisturbed rest between times. Accordingly the very first traumas which can be inflicted upon the helpless infant are a refusal to give him food and comfort when the need for such is indicated, or, conversely, to force food when he is not ready or already had enough. The repetition of such

traumatic situations engenders adverse reactions in both
parent and child, conducive to subsequent difficulties in
the guidance and training of the child.[18]

Dr. Jackson wrote this in 1938. American hospitals have
ignored her warnings for almost forty years, despite growing
clinical evidence which substantiates her opinions.

Child psychiatrist Bruno Bettelheim has explored the
long-range effects of the baby's first feeding experiences. In
his book on infantile autism, Dr. Bettelheim explains how
artificial feeding times contribute to dehumanizing the infant.
Over a twenty-year period, his observations led Dr. Bettelheim to conclude that the most important milestone for a
baby is learning that crying results in his being fed.

If the baby wakes up and screams, and his mother feeds
and soothes him, the baby gets his first experience of trust and
communication. The combined physical satisfaction of
hunger and the emotional security of his mother's prompt
response to his needs gives the baby good feelings about
himself and about other people.[19] This response is so important for the baby that Bettelheim thinks that "nursing and
what happens around it seems to be the nuclear experience
out of which develop all later feelings about oneself and other
persons . . ."

When the newborn infant is separated from his mother
and isolated in a hospital nursery, he is terribly handicapped
in forming this close relationship based on love and need.

> No baby should ever be left to scream with rage and
> fright . . . To a new baby hunger is a terrifying experi-
> ence. Not only is it painful, but he has no knowledge that
> the terror will ever cease.[20]

If the infant cries himself to sleep in the nursery, he may
be too exhausted to nurse well when feeding time finally
arrives. His listless responses to his mother's attempts to feed
him often make the mother feel discouraged, even despair-

ing. In this way, the schedule of the maternity ward robs both mother and baby of their first chance to build a happy relationship.

Each time these frustrations are repeated, the infant "becomes flooded with impotent rage, a helpless victim of inner tensions."[21] Some psychiatrists, such as Erik H. Erikson, hold such upsetting episodes responsible for many later personality disorders. Other mental health professionals explain that repeated nonresponses to the child's earliest needs may make him decide that other people are basically untrustworthy. Since nobody bothers to help him, the child concludes he must not even be worth helping. Overwhelmed by feelings of mistrustfulness and untrustworthiness, the deprived youngster can relate to other people, or develop self-esteem, only with competent professional help.

Bruno Bettelheim pointed out that the damage is not done simply by the hospital's mechanical regulation of the mother-child relationship. Instead, greater harm results because nursery regimentation "prevents the infant from feeling that his actions [crying, smiling] have a significant effect on this important life experience of being fed." When the baby learns that his screams don't bring food, he feels discouraged and demoralized. We might feel half as desperate if we were suddenly dropped into a foreign country and all the inhabitants ignored our pleas for food and water.

One of the world's best-known social anthropologists, Ashley Montagu, says that the opposite of love is not hatred but indifference. Certainly, American society shows true indifference to its newborns' first needs by separating them from their mothers and isolating them in nurseries.

"The removal of the newborn infant to a hospital nursery," states Dr. Montagu, "puts it in an extremely damaging, perilous position. In fact," he adds, "our present American methods of childbirth start human beings off on the wrong foot right from the very first hours of their lives."

Calling the nursery dangerous sounds a bit extreme, but it's well known that babies who are cared for like this indefinitely will die. Child development experts have noted that institutionalized infants often show signs of illness and distress by the time they are just eight weeks old. Because these babies have no chance to form a loving relationship with a person who cares for them, they soon become listless and unhappy; they stop eating. Gradually, the infants lose interest in everything, lose weight, sleep badly, and run a fever. The clinical name for this syndrome is "marasmus" (from the Greek—to waste away). Yet if any one of these babies is taken out of institutional care and placed in a foster home, all the symptoms of "hospitalism" begin to disappear within a day or two.[22]

For the past seventy years, "reports have told consistently about the incredible mortality rate of infants raised in hospitals or institutions . . . under extremely 'sterile' conditions." Why, then, do we continue to allow our newborn babies to be cared for in identical circumstances? The first few postnatal hours and days constitute perhaps the most critical time of the infant's whole life. During such an important period, our babies deserve more humane treatment than they now receive in the typical American hospital.

Besides harming the baby and his mother, our current birth customs shut the father out completely. While the mother gets to enjoy a few brief visits with her baby during feeding times, the father must usually be content with peeks at his new son or daughter through the glass windows of the nursery. The husband may only be permitted short visits, too. When I had my first two children in military hospitals, my husband could only visit for an hour in the afternoon and for another hour in the evening. (No other visitors were allowed.)

To the husband, the days that follow the baby's birth can seem long and lonely. No man looks forward to coming home to an empty house and cooking his own supper. An hour snatched during the afternoon doesn't give the couple much chance to have a satisfactory visit, and the father often must skip the evening visit if he has other children to take care of at home.

These other children in the family also can be innocent victims of our American way of birth. Too frequently, an older child resents the new baby even before he sees it; is it not because of the new baby that his mother suddenly had to go to the hospital?

Even when the older child has been prepared for his mother's absence, he can't help but feel lonely and abandoned while she is in the hospital. And a busy father, preoccupied with concerns for his wife and new baby, often doesn't have the psychological resources to comfort a lonely toddler. The author of *Commonsense Childbirth* spoke for many women when she described her loneliness for her older son during the hospital birth of her second baby. Hearing his "sad little voice over the phone" stirred her anger against the hospital rule that kept children out of the maternity ward.

It ought to be obvious that "childbirth is a family affair, everyone in the family being strongly affected by its outcome."[23] Yet our maternity care system neglects the most basic needs of every member of the family. The conventional style of American delivery is traumatic for the mother and dangerous for her baby. It excludes the father and fans the sparks of sibling rivalry. Instead of uniting all its members to share in a major family event, our American way of birth separates, divides, and weakens every family that endures it.

NOTES

1. William J. Cromie, "Drunken Roosters Aid in Motherhood Study," *The Sacramento Union*, January 16, 1974, A 12.
2. H.M.I. Liley, M.D., and Beth Day, *Modern Motherhood* (New York: Random House, 1969), p. 75.

3. Deborah Tanzer and Jean L. Block, *Why Natural Childbirth?* (Garden City, N.Y.: Doubleday & Co., 1972), p. 58.
4. Geraldine Lux Flanagan, *The First Nine Months of Life* (New York: Simon & Schuster, 1962), p. 88.
5. T. Berry Brazelton, M.D., "What Childbirth Drugs Can Do To Your Child," *Redbook,* February 1971, p. 146.
6. "Testing Baby's Brain," *Newsweek,* June 11, 1973, p. 116.
7. Barbara Seaman, *Free and Female* (New York: Coward, McCann & Geoghegan, Inc., 1972), p. 151.
8. Helen Wessel, *Natural Childbirth and the Family* (New York: Harper & Row, 1973), p. 81.
9. Stephanie Caruana, "Childbirth for the Joy of It," *Playgirl,* March 1974, p. 55.
10. Deborah Tanzer and Jean L. Block, op. cit., p. 54-55.
11. Virginia Apgar and Joan Beck, *Is My Baby All Right?* (New York: Trident Press, 1972), p. 119.
12. The Boston Children's Medical Center, *Pregnancy, Birth and the Newborn Baby* (Boston: Boston Children's Medical Center, 1971), p. 278.
13. Constance A. Bean, *Methods of Childbirth* (Garden City, N.Y.: Doubleday & Company, 1972), p. 132.
14. Ibid., p. 136.
15. Erwin Di Cyan, "Hospital Germs—Why They're Extra Deadly," *Family Weekly,* October 7, 1972, p. 25.
16. Nancy Stoller Shaw, *Forced Labor* (Elmsford, N.Y.: Pergamon Press Inc., 1974), pp. 120-121.
17. Herbert Thoms, M.D., *Understanding Natural Childbirth* (New York: McGraw-Hill Book Company, Inc., 1950), p. 109.
18. Ibid.
19. Bruno Bettelheim, M.D., *The Empty Fortress: Infantile Autism and the Birth of the Self* (New York: The Free Press, 1967), p. 25.
20. Sheila Kitzinger, *The Experience of Childbirth* (New York: Taplinger Publishing Company, 1962), p. 235.
21. Bruno Bettelheim, op. cit., p. 19.
22. Niles Newton, M.D., *Maternal Emotions* (New York: Paul E. Hoeber, Inc., 1955), pp. 63-64.
23. Lester Dessez Hazell, *Commonsense Childbirth* (New York: G.P. Putnam's Sons, 1969), xxxv.

OTHER SOURCES

Irwin Chabon, M.D., *Awake and Aware* (New York: Delacorte Press, 1966), p. 30.
"Why Can't Mothers Deliver Their Babies at Home?" *The Sacramento Union,* May 5, 1974, E9.

Sheldon H. Cherry, M.D., *Understanding Pregnancy and Childbirth* (Indianapolis: Bobbs-Merrill, 1973), p. 60.

Howard R. and Martha E. Lewis, *The Medical Offenders* (New York: Simon & Schuster, 1970), p. 212.

Robert A. Bradley, M.D., *Husband-Coached Childbirth* (New York: Harper & Row, 1965), p. 176.

Ashley Montagu, appearing on *The Tonight Show*, November 16, 1973, interviewed by Johnny Carson on NBC.

Suzanne Arms, "How Hospitals Complicate Childbirth," *Ms.*, May 1975.

4

ALTERNATIVES TO THE HOSPITAL

Do all American hospitals practice the reactionary birth procedures described in the past chapters? By no means. Today, enlightened and humane birth customs can be found in many American cities.

The hospitals in Denver, Colorado, for example, have been heavily influenced by the crusade of Dr. Robert A. Bradley, author of *Husband-Coached Childbirth.* As a result, Denver couples can stay together during childbirth, and nobody forces drugs or anesthesia upon the mother. She may deliver her baby in a comfortable squatting position, with her husband supporting her back. After the birth, the new parents themselves usually carry their newborn baby out of the delivery room.

West Park Hospital in Los Angeles lets the mother skip the predelivery drugs and shave. She and her husband spend the first part of labor in a private, darkened room; they go to a quiet delivery room for the birth. The woman does not have to put her legs in stirrups, nor are her hands tied. West Park's maternity program appeared in the news in 1974, when actor Donald Sutherland took Francine Recette there for the birth of their baby.

Very few hospitals, however, allow their clients as much freedom as the Booth Maternity Center in Philadelphia. There the mother literally runs her own birth, much as she would do at home. Her pubic hair is not routinely shaved; she is not forced to have an enema. She receives pain-killing drugs only if she wants them, not when a doctor or nurse decides she needs them. During labor, she can walk around the hospital; her husband can be with her at all times. When the birth occurs, it does not have to happen on a delivery table or be preceded by an episiotomy. The mother is allowed to push her baby out slowly, rather than having a doctor drag it out with forceps.

Allowing the *mother* to control these circumstances of childbirth is truly revolutionary, since most American hospitals give all such authority to the *doctor*.

> The doctor is director—he makes all the important decisions in the delivery room. This practice is supported legally and institutionally. The doctor decides the kind of anesthesia to be used, the amount and kind of drugs, the timing for the birth, whether to use forceps and what type is best, the use of episiotomy, and the positioning of the patient. All this is justified by the fact that the doctor does the delivery, and therefore has the right to decide *how* it will be done.[1]

No known American institution yet follows the example set by Nesbitt Memorial Hospital in Kingston, Pennsylvania. There, patients of obstetrics chief William Hazlett take classes where they learn natural childbirth techniques. During the delivery, Dr. Hazlett stands by—*while the husbands deliver their own babies!*

During the past seven years, over one thousand fathers have delivered their own babies at Nesbitt Memorial. But some of the do-it-yourself deliveries have also taken place in Dr. Hazlett's office across the street. If the parents go to the hospital, however, the wife is not put on an uncomfortable delivery table; the baby can be born in a regular room. The father is not required to wear a surgical gown, mask, gloves, or foot coverings, either.

"There has been talk of the lack of sterile control in a hospital room," admits Dr. Hazlett, "but we've proved that there are no more germs there than in the delivery room."[2]

How do parents like the idea of delivering their own children? So much so that some of them have switched doctors and traveled from other cities to have their babies this way.

"There's nothing on earth like it," beamed a young construction worker who delivered his baby daughter under Dr. Hazlett's supervision.

"I wouldn't have it any other way than this, now," declared a wife who had her first two children delivered by doctors, and her third baby delivered by her husband.

"None of the fathers crumple in the corner," testifies an obstetrics supervisor at Nesbitt Memorial. In fact, most of the fathers make good midwives. In 1974 a national newspaper ran a picture story about Dr. Hazlett; one father was shown clamping and cutting his newborn daughter's umbilical cord, while Dr. Hazlett stood in the background. (The week after this story appeared, the paper received hundreds of letters from readers. Almost unanimously, they approved of the fathers' delivering the babies and pointed out how such births could help unify the family.)

If hospitals are now becoming this progressive, why do more and more couples still want home childbirth? One of the biggest reasons is that, despite a gradual softening in American maternity-ward policies, very few hospitals have offered parents enough control of the birth process. According to neonatologist Stanley Graven, the few changes many hospitals *have* made may be quite superficial; although they may allow the husband to stay with his wife during labor, the underlying philosophy remains the same, and the quality of maternity care does not improve much.

This forces couples into making some unwelcome decisions if they want hospital care. For example, they may want to go to a hospital that encourages husband-coached childbirth. But what if the wife must also accept fetal monitoring and an episiotomy? Once young parents find out that the hospital insists on a glucose I.V., supplemental oxygen, and a lying-down, legs-tied delivery position, they may decide that this version of natural childbirth is not quite "natural" enough for them.

An example of what some institutions consider to be an ideal family-centered childbirth was presented on "Birth and Babies," a 1974 ABC television special. Viewers were introduced to a young California couple; we saw them attending prenatal classes, practicing natural childbirth exercises. We also saw the husband in the delivery room, properly masked and gowned. Later, we observed the couple participating in the hospital's family-centered care program, feeding their baby together.

A beautiful picture of natural childbirth? Many viewers disagreed. The mother had received an epidural anesthetic, and the baby was subjected to fetal monitoring. When it came time to deliver the baby, the mother couldn't push it out fast enough, so the anesthesiologist shoved from above her abdomen while the obstetrician pulled with what looked like a vacuum extractor. During the delivery, the anesthesiologist clapped a mask over the mother's face; they told her she needed it because she was hyperventilating.

It was hard to see what was "natural" about such a birth, from the mother's point of view. Even worse, I thought, was the baby's condition. She was born quite limp and purple. After aspirating her a few times, she cried a bit, and the doctor presented her to her mother.

"There you are," he declared proudly, "a beautiful baby girl."

The obstetrician's congratulations proved to be slightly premature. When he handed the baby to her mother, it collapsed into a bluish, unresponsive heap. Quickly, the doctor snatched her up again. This time he worked with the aspirator until the infant was breathing on her own.

Although the baby was laid right on the mother, she was not allowed to touch or hold it. Instead, the doctor repeatedly told her to keep her hands under the sterile drapes. Finally, the baby was moved to a small incubator, where she was left, naked, to scream pitifully. Nobody made any effort to wrap her up, or to hold and comfort her.

To me, this illustrates how completely the hospital delivery atmosphere robs parents of control during the birth of their own babies. Even a family-centered birth in one of the nation's best hospitals is so mechanized and routinized that nobody has time to meet the baby's first needs. The mother cannot be allowed to touch her baby, lest she contaminate the "sterile field." The father usually doesn't dare to touch the baby at this early stage, and the doctor must turn his attention to the afterbirth and episiotomy. Meanwhile, the naked newborn lies in a corner, screaming her poor little head off.

If today's American parents don't want to participate in scenes like this, what alternatives do they have? *Commonsense Childbirth* proposes that mothers have their babies in "Maternity Motels" instead of hospitals. These institutions would serve only maternity cases, thus avoiding many of the hospital-acquired infections which plague so many babies in this country. A woman who visited the Maternity Motel would see one team of midwives, nurses, doctors, physiotherapists and mother's helpers. The team would get to know not only the expectant mother, but also her husband and children. The Maternity Motel's baby-sitting nursery would also care for her children during checkups and later, when she went into labor.

When the mother checked into the Maternity Motel to have her baby, her husband could come right along with her and stay in her room. During early labor, the couple could order from the restaurant's menu or visit the cocktail lounge. Television lounges and game rooms would also help labor to pass quickly. When it was time for the baby to be born, the parents could return to their motel room, where the baby could be born in bed. If the delivery proceeded normally, it could be assisted by a nurse-midwife. After the birth, however, she would leave the family alone to enjoy the new baby together.

When the couple felt tired, the father could carry the baby down to the nursery for the night, so a nurse could watch him. During the day, baby would return to the parents' room; older brothers and sisters could visit him as much as they wish. Since the Maternity Motel functions like a luxury hotel, appointments with a masseuse and hairdresser could be scheduled when the mother wants them. Because the Maternity Motel also provides the best obstetrical care, sessions with a physiotherapist would be scheduled so that the mother could get started on a postnatal exercise program.

The author of *Commonsense Childbirth* proposed this plan not just as a utopian pipe dream. As a cultural anthropologist, she studied childbirth customs all over the world. During her research, she collected "the best features of many obstetrical hospitals from several countries."[3] Then she incorporated these features into her description of the ideal Maternity Motel. (Her remarkable proposition can be read in full in "The Choice Is Ours," a chapter in *Commonsense Childbirth*.)

It is now over six years since Mrs. Hazell's book was published, and Maternity Motels haven't exactly been springing up all over the country. In 1975, however, New York City's Maternity Center Association established a demonstration project to provide satisfying care for low-risk expectant mothers. Featuring labor and delivery in a homelike atmosphere, the project offers prenatal education, delivery by nurse-midwives, and home visits following the birth of the baby. The project also includes supervision by obstetricians, and a pediatric examination for the newborn baby. Like all of the Maternity Center's services, the cost for each birth is kept as low as possible.

Another feature of Mrs. Hazell's maternity ideal has been

incorporated at Scripps Hospital in La Jolla, California, where older brothers and sisters may visit the obstetrics ward to see the newborn baby. By appointment, they are escorted to an isolated viewing room where their mothers join them. Together they can look through a glass window into the nursery. Although this ceremonial routine may sound ridiculous to mothers who have had their babies at home, it is really a step forward. Without a doubt, if it were widely adopted, this innovation would ease much of the strain on families who must bear their children in American hospitals.

Parents who live beyond the range of these few programs, though, usually face a hard choice. They must either accept the welter of technology in our hospitals or have their babies at home.

Women in other parts of the world do not have to confront this difficult decision, for other countries approach hospital childbirth much more humanely. A South African mother, for example, may well prefer to have her baby in the hospital, in order to use its decompression suit. Operating on the same principle as a "baby bubble," this suit lifts the abdomen away from the uterus during each contraction. As a result of the decrease of pressure on the contracting uterus, it can work more effectively and the mother is freed from uterine pain.[4] When the decompression suit is used during labor, pain-relieving drugs are almost never needed. The birth occurs naturally, but in less time than conventional deliveries.

Natural birth in shorter time also results from an imaginative innovation being used in Eskilstuna, Sweden. Central Hospital's chief of obstetrics, Dr. Sune Dahlgren, uses a Japanese-made cervical vibrator up to three times during first stage labor. When the vibrator is applied to the cervix between contractions, it helps the cervix relax, which makes it work more effectively. The resulting deliveries take place in approximately half the normal time. Yet, once again, birth proceeds normally and naturally.

Although Dr. Dahlgren's book on vibrator-assisted deliveries was not yet published at the time this was written, he was kind enough to make his preliminary report available. After studying the data on several hundred Swedish deliveries—both conventional and vibrator-assisted, he published these conclusions:

> The method has positive effects on both mother and child and also for the delivering staff. It can be looked upon as a new approach to the problem of pain relief during labor, where the individual labor-pain will not be affected, but their number will be greatly reduced—the method is, so to speak, labor-saving. The mother will not be so tired, and there will also be psychological advantages. The child will not be so long in delivery, and the trauma against the fetal head seems to diminish. The method saves much time for the staff, and deliveries can be completed in office-time. No complications have hitherto occurred and the method seems to be without side effects.[5]

One of the most famous foreign birth innovations in recent years comes from France. In Paris, obstetrician Frederick Leboyer has delivered over one thousand babies with his "gentle-birth" method. With lights turned low and in a quiet atmosphere, he eases the baby onto the mother's stomach so she can hold him. Unlike most obstetricians, Dr. Leboyer does not suction the baby's breathing passages immediately. Instead, he waits a few moments, so that the baby continues to receive oxygen through the umbilical cord. When the cord stops pulsating, he cuts it; then he immerses the baby in a warm bath for a few minutes to help it relax and recover from the upsetting birth experience.

According to Dr. Leboyer, the conventional method of birth is a "barbaric way to bring babies into the world."[6]

"Babies are terrorized . . . their first minutes on earth are a private hell," he maintains. Dr. Leboyer thinks newborn babies scream with fear when they are born, and that the delivery room atmosphere and procedures increase this trauma. Accordingly, he does away with glaring lights, loud voices, suctioning devices and such practices as holding the baby up by its feet and slapping it.

French mothers who have borne their babies his way say that Dr. Leboyer's method produces happier babies. For one thing, the infants visibly lose their tension in the bath. Once they have calmed down, they usually smile, and they may even begin to babble—all during the first ten minutes of their lives. And years later, their postnatal self-confidence remains. Parents of seven- and eight-year-old children who were born via the "gentle-birth" method say that they are happier, more relaxed, and less afraid of life than their children who were born conventionally.[7]

Another study of fifty Leboyer-delivered children discovered the same things. In addition, the Sorbonne child psychologist in charge of this survey discovered such phenomena as higher intelligence and earlier interest in the world and people.

"There is no question in my mind, these children *are* noticeably different from others who were delivered in the 'classical' way," observes Dr. Danielle Rapoport.

Of hospital deliveries in another foreign country—Spain—I've had firsthand experience. My husband was stationed near Madrid when we were expecting our third baby. After a traumatic delivery at the base hospital the year before, we searched for a good Spanish doctor to deliver the next one at home. Finally we found an obstetrician who had many English-speaking patients. As a father of eight children, he was sympathetic to the needs of both mother and baby and sensitive to the dangers of common delivery analgesics. Although Dr. Chiva agreed to deliver the baby at home, he thought we should consider having it at the private hospital where he practiced.

When we learned what the Clinica Santa Elena was like,

we had the baby there. Operated by Catholic nuns, it offered beautiful private rooms—each with a full bath, terrace, and fold-out couch for the husband to sleep on. The baby stayed in the room, too; around midnight one of the sisters came and wheeled the bassinette down to the nursery so the parents could get a full night's sleep.

During the day, anyone could come and visit—including children. The day after little Milagros was born, she had five visitors. Her older sisters loved being able to touch her and hold her tiny hand, especially since they had expected to be barred from the hospital completely.

In addition to the obstetrician, nurses and the nuns, we had a wonderful Spanish midwife. She arrived at the hospital shortly after we did, stayed with us throughout labor, and assisted with the delivery. Then she washed and dressed the newborn baby and filled out the papers for the birth certificate. Each day she would return to chat with us and to check on the baby. As I remember, her fee for all these services was only twenty-five dollars!

Dr. Chiva, the obstetrician, charged only seventy-five dollars. His fee included all the prenatal office visits and a postnatal checkup. The hospital bill came to less than a hundred dollars for a three-day stay. This seemed very modest, especially considering the *five* delicious meals they served every day.

What I appreciated most about this hospital, however, was the absence of technological intrusions. Fetal monitoring, I.V. setups, oxygen, blood tests, vaginal and rectal examinations, temperature and blood-pressure routines were almost completely neglected. (The nuns did take my temperature once or twice, apologizing as they did so!) In spite of the absence of hospital technological aids, the Spanish mothers looked just as healthy and seemed a lot happier than their American counterparts.

Their babies appeared to get along very well, too. One of

the nursery sisters let me visit the baby room, or "nest" as they call it in Spanish, after the babies had been settled for the night. The infants looked alert, but contented. Not one of the thirty-odd babies screamed or cried—either because the nuns cuddled them when they fussed, or because they spent sixteen hours daily with their own parents. It was quite a contrast to the average American newborn nursery, where each baby screams for almost two hours a day.[8]

One mother told a home birth seminar in Santa Cruz, California, that for four-hour periods she would stand outside the nursery window in tears, watching her infant son cry continuously. She described this experience as the most painful event in her life. Yet her delivery took place in a San Francisco hospital famous for its progressive maternity practices!

In the United States today, expectant parents must usually choose between the present panoply of technology in the hospital or no medical help at all during childbirth. Furthermore, it's even harder to consider a home delivery when so many doctors criticize it so loudly.

"Taking the risk of home birth is like playing Russian roulette," declares obstetrician Robert Bradley. But since Dr. Bradley has done so much to awaken Americans to the dangers of childbirth drugs, he also admits that some women might have to take this very risk—if they are unfortunate enough to live in "some small woebegone town without a humanistically inclined hospital."[9]

Since Dr. Bradley practices in Denver, where every hospital has a progressive obstetrics program—(thanks to him!)—it's easy for him to assume that only hospitals in small towns have problems meeting the needs of their maternity patients. The true picture, however, doesn't match this assumption. Even in such "liberated" areas as the San Fernando Valley and the San Francisco Bay area in California, natural childbirth may only be offered by one-quarter to one-third of all hospitals. And in the Washington, D.C. area, over half of the hospitals surveyed still didn't admit husbands to the delivery room by the early 1970s.

Dr. Bradley advocates consumer resistance to such policies.

"Obstetrics hospitals that do not open their delivery room doors to husbands and that do not practice humanistic obstetrics should go broke after a while because people simply won't go there," asserts Bradley.

In order to promote such changes in hospital policy, parents and doctors have formed several organizations. The American Society for Psychoprophylaxis in Obstetrics (ASPO) and the International Childbirth Education Association (ICEA) are two of them. Although the emphasis may vary, most such educational groups direct their efforts toward either "prepared" or "family-centered" childbirth. Prepared childbirth simply means the parents have attended from six to eight prenatal classes; family-centered childbirth goes a step further and allows the husband to stand by his wife in the delivery room.

Both of these modes of birth stop short of "natural" childbirth, which was introduced by Dr. Grantly Dick-Read in the 1930s. It means birth without anesthetics, and usually without pain-relieving drugs, too. Although the majority of American obstetricians oppose natural childbirth, the Bradley-method classes in husband-coached childbirth advocate it. The increasing popularity of the Bradley method of natural childbirth bodes well for American babies who will be born during the next decade.

If couples can't find an obstetrician who practices true natural childbirth, they may then consider having their baby at home. Although most Americans feel that this would be taking a terrible chance, statistics say otherwise. For example, one borough in London, England, recorded a recent 800 home births with absolutely no infant or maternal deaths. Another borough boasted 1,500 home deliveries with only 2 stillbirths.[10] (The same number of hospital deliveries in California would result in an infant mortality toll of approximately 35.)

Since England has a medically supervised system of home delivery, however, it might seem unfair to compare their home births to American home births, which usually occur completely outside the medical system. As the surge in American childbirth at home is so recent, reliable statistics are hard to find, but since 1971, midwives in Northern California have delivered almost three hundred babies at home with only one infant death. When the midwives brought this baby to a doctor for emergency treatment, they learned that he suffered from a congenital abnormality which would have been fatal even if he had been born in a hospital.

Out of approximately five hundred recent doctor-supervised home births in the Point Reyes area of California, results have been equally good.

"We don't know of any instances where a life has been lost that might have been saved had the birth taken place in a hospital," reports Dr. Wesley Sokolosky. "We've had no maternal deaths," he adds.

Once again it would appear that these home deliveries had a record that was almost five times better than hospital deliveries in the same state. (Out of every 300 births in California hospitals, about 4 babies die.) Also, the home delivery statistics supplied by midwives and physicians do *not* include those babies who are born at home without their assistance. Still another group of babies are born at home with no medical help; no birth certificate is ever filed, either. If the numbers of these two groups of home-delivered babies were added to the totals delivered by midwives and doctors, the home-birth safety record might be even more impressive.

Besides having a better chance of surviving the birth, a home-born baby runs less risk of picking up a disease or infection from a germ-filled hospital. This danger has risen dramatically since the government prohibited the use of the antibacterial hexachlorophene in hospital's centralized new-born nurseries.[11]

Consumers now seem to be more aware of such risks. A California couple who live on a Yolo County farm recently decided to have their first baby at home. One of their main reasons was the prevalence of disease in all hospitals. Another reason was their distrust of drugs given to the mother which they realize can reach the unborn baby in a very short time. A third reason offered by these young people was their unwillingness to have the mother strapped into a delivery position they regard as both dangerous and agonizing.[12]

"We want to have total control over the birth of our child and want to be together from labor through postdelivery in an environment that doesn't treat you as if you are sick," they explain.

"Most of our friends have also had healthy home births," adds the wife. She saw a midwife-assisted home delivery about a year ago, which helped to bolster her confidence in her own natural abilities.

Home births are coming to be preferred not only by such young "back-to-nature" couples but often by some from the middle and upper classes as well. Although doctors frequently dismiss couples who plan to have their babies at home as freaks or hippies, professionals who work with these parents say that they usually show a "high level of education, combined with great interest in the physiological and psychological aspects of childbearing."[13]

"About half of the people I see are 'hip,' " reports Nancy Mills, a midwife who attends home births in Santa Rosa, California. "Another fourth are well educated and concerned with aesthetics. And the remaining fourth are extremely strong in their religious affirmations and have chosen home birth for spiritual reasons."[14]

When the British Association for Improvement of Maternity Services conducted a wide-ranging survey, they discovered some surprising opinions. Of the English mothers who had experienced both home and hospital deliveries, *fully 84 percent preferred childbirth at home!*[15]

Some of the reasons for the popularity of home births in England were explained in a *Saturday Evening Post* article by Susan Eisenhower Bradshaw, one of President Eisenhower's four grandchildren. Her 1971 marriage to a British lawyer and their subsequent move to London paved the way for her introduction to childbirth at home, English style. According to Mrs. Bradshaw, this is why British mothers continue to prefer home childbirth:

> Nine-to-five inductions for doctors' convenience are becoming more common. "Rooming in" for the baby doesn't exist in many hospitals. Husbands are still denied the right to see their own baby's birth. Younger children are denied access to their mothers during hospitalization and are forced to meet their newest "rival" at the doorstep. Anesthetics are encouraged and even pushed in some instances, despite the wishes of the mother.[16]

In her article, Mrs. Bradshaw described the hospital birth of her first baby as gratifying, but the labor that preceded it was exasperating. Not only did she have to cope with her contractions, but the doctor kept coming in and urging her to accept analgesia.

"Doctor knows best, let me give you something for the pain," he repeated, in spite of the fact that she neither wanted nor needed it.

"Don't listen to what they taught you at those silly classes, I really know best."

Mothers who have their babies in hospitals this side of the Atlantic may experience the same difficulties. In 1974, a friend of mine had her baby at the University of California Medical Center in San Francisco.

"They really try to push their drugs," she reported.

"We felt they didn't like us because we knew too much," added her young husband.

This couple had prepared for a natural childbirth. They had attended the full program of prenatal classes together, and the husband had remained with his wife throughout the delivery. Furthermore, she had an unexpectedly short, easy labor. Yet the hospital staff were affronted because the wife didn't want the drugs they offered.

"I have seen some attending nurses, even interns, and especially anesthetists who by their facial expressions and attitudes show they resent a mother giving birth without their medication," stated Dr. Robert Bradley in *Husband-Coached Childbirth.* Ten years later, these attitudes remain largely unchanged.

According to *Our Bodies, Ourselves,* medical personnel are trained to deal with sick patients; they often do not know how to handle normal people who have a sense of entitlement.[17] As a result, when a patient wants to have a baby *her* way, the hospital staff may label her as aggressive, uptight, or a time waster. The woman who insists on her right to natural childbirth should expect to be considered a difficult patient, or even a troublemaker, by nurses and doctors.

"Postpartum blues may be exaggerated by hospitalization and isolation with interruption of natural social processes," theorizes Dr. Robert S. Spitzer, a California doctor who has attended many home deliveries. He thinks that having a baby at home seems to markedly lower the high incidence of postnatal depression found after hospital deliveries.[18]

Natural Childbirth and the Family places the blame for postpartum depression more squarely upon the American way of birth. According to this book, a natural birth provides an opportunity for the mother to experience the physical and emotional climax of her pregnancy. Without being awake and going through this "peak experience," the woman cannot experience the resulting sense of release and relief after her baby is born.

> This climax is essential. A mother who has missed it and had a passive, frigid birth, due to anesthetics, local injec-

tions, or hypnosis, still is emotionally in a state of expectancy. She looks at her child, but experiences no euphoria, no sense of exhilaration. But a release from pent-up emotion must come! If an adequate birth climax does not provide it, it will come later, in spells of frustrated weeping, like the tantrums of the small child who cannot explain, and indeed does not know, what it is he wants.[19]

Experiments with animals have shown that this line of thinking rests on solid ground. When a herd of wild deer was observed over a fifteen-year period, no doe refused to accept and nurture her fawn. But when six pregnant does were anesthetized during labor, *each of the six refused to accept her own newborn fawn* when she awoke after the birth.[20]

Separating mother and baby right after birth has had similar upsetting effects in both humans and animals. When newborn goats, calves, and lambs were removed from their mothers right after birth and later returned to them, the mothers pushed them away and sometimes even attacked them. If the mothers kept their babies for four days before the separation, however, they accepted their babies when they were returned.

It has been suggested that humans follow similar behavior patterns. Several studies have shown that premature babies who had to be separated from their mothers and specially cared for during their first few weeks of life may later suffer terrible consequences. Between 25 percent and 40 percent of our battered children have spent their first few weeks of life hospitalized in a nursery for premature infants. Apparently, after the immediate separation following birth, their mothers were simply unable to form the normal emotional bonds with their babies.

One of the biggest cases for home birth is the unity it gives to the family, the sense of togetherness parents feel when they work together to deliver a baby that they have conceived together. Whatever misgivings an individual parent may harbor before the home birth of a baby, afterwards they are unanimous: having a baby at home made them more of a "family."

"Anyone who has helped his wife deliver their baby—helped her through the hard work—has just partaken of the greatest miracle allowed man by his Creator. What a togetherness!" This is what Dan Skowronski, of Cleveland Heights, Ohio, thinks of home childbirth. He should know. He delivered his fourth child at home, making a tape recording of the birth. Leaving the recorder on, he awoke his three older children so they could welcome their new little sister. Their "ooohs" and delighted comments are all on tape.

Mr. Skowronski's mother-in-law "nearly had a fit" about their planned home delivery. But when she heard the tape, her feelings changed.

"She nearly cried," recalls Dan. "I think she finally understood why we wanted this so much."

Hospital technology can never substitute for the comfort of one's own bed, say most mothers who have had their babies at home. The privacy afforded by remaining in one's own home helps the mother avoid the unnecessary embarrassment she often suffers in the hospital. Anxiety and fear can raise the mother's blood pressure and increase the severity of her pains. At home, however, she can relax when and where she wants. Long before her contractions start to feel unbearable, she can fix herself a soothing drink. Sipping bourbon and ginger ale tastes better than having Demerol and glucose I.V.s in the hospital, and it works better, too, say women who have tried both during labor.

"I'd rather take my 'chances' at home than subject myself to man-made misery," explained a Salt Lake City registered nurse who had her fourth baby at home. "A natural, intentionally unattended birth is a delightful, exhilarating, tremendously satisfying experience. It is spiritually ennobling, in contrast to the institutional experience, which is often degrading, discouraging, and even downright distasteful."

How great is the probability that something may go

wrong during a home birth? One physician I queried said that for a woman with a history of previous normal births, who is well motivated and receives good prenatal care, the risks are less than one percent. That is, a mother with good obstetrical history has a better than 99 percent chance of having her baby at home with no problems. This does not, however, rule out the possibility of having first babies at home, too. The pros and cons of doing this will be covered in a later chapter.

Another doctor mentioned a little-discussed reason for the growing popularity of childbirth at home. If the baby is born at home, its parents can share in making decisions about its resuscitation, should it be badly malformed. In hospitals, on the other hand, the staff who attends the delivery may be trained to make the baby start breathing before evaluating its condition or forming a prognosis. When the mother wakes up, she may learn that her baby did not breathe for half an hour and is now being kept alive by a breathing machine. At this point, it's too late for the parents to tell the doctors not to resuscitate their baby if it doesn't respond to natural, nonheroic methods of inducing respiration.

Some miracles of modern science have led to tragedy. One little boy was kept alive until he was eighteen months old, when doctors gave up; they were unable to reconstruct enough of his small intestine so that he could eat. Faced with the possibility of raising a son who could never eat or drink, the parents decided to remove the artificial supports that had kept him alive and growing for over a year.

In 1974, a severely deformed baby was born at Portland's Maine Medical Center. The baby's esophagus did not connect to his stomach, so he could not eat. He had no left eye. His left ear canal was missing. Doctors guessed that he might never be able to see, hear or speak; there was a question as to whether the baby would ever gain consciousness. Even if subjected to corrective operations, the physicians estimated that the baby would still be "severely palsied, blind, deaf, and unable to communicate."

The baby's parents refused permission for corrective

surgery since the pediatrician advised them it would probably do no good, anyway. But a Superior Court judge ordered the operation after the medical center sued the parents. While lawyers for both sides were threatening to take the case to Maine's Supreme Court, the baby died.

Emotionally, the two parents were shattered by the experience. It was bad enough to have had a newborn baby with such distressing deformities; what made it worse was that the parents so completely lost control of the birth. Instead of acting like responsible adults, they became pawns in a legal battle. For in spite of the fact that both parents and doctors agreed the baby faced a marginally human life—a life which would be filled with suffering—a judge stepped in and ordered the operation. (The parents weren't the only ones who were confused; the medical center had considered financing their appeal to the Supreme Court, so it could obtain a definitive ruling on such cases for the future.)[21]

"They [the parents] were most disturbed by the actions of the court in divesting them of the right to make an intimate parental decision that they believe was rightfully theirs," said the couple's lawyer.

The mother and father added a further thought.

"Since nature determined that this infant was not a viable life, it was the court and not the parents that played God in deciding that the infant should be kept alive contrary to the laws of nature."

To a couple who wants to have their child born as naturally as possible, such examples serve as fearful warnings of not only the power of medical technology but also of the possibility of governmental intrusion.

Increasing numbers of young people today don't want to allow hospitals to force life into their defective babies and then drop the problem of sustaining that life in the parents' laps. Many couples feel that since they wouldn't want to prolong life artificially when they are ready to die, they would not want a doctor to *induce* life artificially if their baby does not respond to normal measures. Yet they don't trust the hospitals to go along with their decision. Many of them hesitate to discuss the question with their obstetrician, perhaps out of a superstitious fear that talking about such possibilities may bring bad luck. And in the face of the widespread assumption that doctors always work to preserve life, such couples may also be afraid of being misunderstood or thought of as "heartless."

So home birth often ends up as the only way open to parents who want certain choices, yet feel unable to get them in the hospital. Many couples then turn to home delivery almost by default.

"The hospital experience terrifies us," they admit. "Their way of birth disgusts us. So we will have our baby at home."

Most couples who are conscientious enough to assume this great responsibility are also responsible enough to be very much afraid of the risks connected with home delivery.

What exactly are those risks? Do parents really have to approach home childbirth with fear and trembling? The next chapter will look for realistic answers to these questions.

NOTES

1. Nancy Stoller Shaw, *Forced Labor: Maternity Care in the United States* (Elmsford, N.Y.: Pergamon Press Inc., 1974), p. 85.
2. Peter Bridge, "1,000 Midwife Dads Do It Themselves," *National Star*, November 9, 1974, p. 12.
3. Lester Dessez Hazell, *Commonsense Childbirth* (New York: G.P. Putnam's Sons, 1969), p. 180.
4. H.M.I. Liley, M.D. and Beth Day, *Modern Motherhood* (New York: Random House, 1969), p. 63.
5. Sune Dahlgren, "Reduction of Delivery Time by Cervical Dilatation Induced by Vibrations," *IRCS*, November 1973, (73-11) 22-13-7.
6. Tereska Torres, "From Womb to World," *Ms.*, July 1974, p. 22.
7. Ibid.
8. Helen Wessel, *Natural Childbirth and the Family* (New York: Harper & Row, 1973), p. 245.

9. Stephanie Caruana,"Childbirth For the Joy of It," *Playgirl*, March 1974, p. 55.
10. Susan Eisenhower Bradshaw, "Two Jam Jars, One Bucket, Two Pudding Basins," (Home Birth, a Personal Account), *The Saturday Evening Post,* May 1974, p. 96.
11. Erwin Di Cyan, "Hospital Germs—Why They're Extra Deadly," *Family Weekly,* October 7, 1973, p. 25.
12. Hilary Abramson, "Why Can't Mothers Deliver Their Babies at Home?" *The Sacramento Union,* Sunday, May 5, 1974, E8.
13. "New Demonstration Project Planned," *Special Delivery* (Maternity Center Association Newsletter) Autumn 1974, p. 5.
14. Kaye Yost, "At Home Or in the Hospital?" *California Living,* November 3, 1974, p. 10.
15. Susan Eisenhower Bradshaw, op. cit., p. 96.
16. Ibid.
17. Boston Women's Health Book Collective, Inc., *Our Bodies, Ourselves* (New York: Simon & Schuster, 1973), p. 243.
18. Raven Lang, *Birth Book* (Ben Lomond, California: Genesis Press, 1972).
19. Wessel, op. cit., p. 224.
20. Ibid., p. 222.
21. "Infant's Father Unsure About Future Action," *Portland Times,* February 25, 1974, p. 1.

OTHER SOURCES
(listed as they appear in text)

Donald Sutherland, "Childbirth Is Not for Mothers Only," *Ms.,* May 1974, p. 47.
Elliott H. McCleary, *New Miracles of Childbirth,* (New York: David McKay Company, 1974).
Jay Nelson Tuck, "Make Room for Daddy," (Medifacts), *Women's Day,* October 1972, p. 42.
"Tots Visit Maternity Ward," *The Sacramento Bee,* August 14, 1974, p. D1.
Steven Englund, " 'Birth Without Violence'," *The New York Times Magazine,* December 8, 1974.
Interview with Three Midwives, Santa Rosa, California, December 11, 1973.
Kaye Yost, "At Home Or In The Hospital?" *California Living,* November 3, 1974.
Robert A. Bradley, M.D., *Husband-Coached Childbirth* (New York: Harper & Row, 1965).
Jean McCann, "They Want to Have Their Babies at Home," *Marriage,* June 1971.

5

WHAT ARE THE RISKS?

"So home delivery is more natural. The birth will be easier for my wife and safer for the baby. Having the baby at home will be far more natural; it will be more private, more human, and less expensive. We'll be able to share the responsibility for making important decisions about our baby. But will a home birth be safe? And is it legal?"

These questions must be faced by the couple thinking about childbirth at home. Before contemplating home delivery more seriously, both parents owe it to themselves to consider all the various risks involved. Not only may the need for medical attention arise during labor, for example, but legal and social complications should be considered.

Outside of the few American communities where home birth has gained increased acceptance, the very mention of it causes negative reactions. Couples who announce that they are considering delivering their baby at home ought to expect anything from raised eyebrows to outright hostility from their friends, relatives, and neighbors. Having a baby at home is definitely not for the thin-skinned.

In *Commonsense Childbirth,* Lester D. Hazell describes the

attitude parents must face if they want to have their baby at home.

"Our strange society will not hold it against you if your baby is palsied or has his intelligence stunted by too much anesthesia in the hospital, but if he is born at home with a birthmark or a club foot, the fault will be called yours."[1]

When they encountered skeptical questions, one California couple defended their choice of home delivery as the more responsible of their alternatives. They decided their unborn baby would have a much better start on life if the mother could avoid the drugs and unnatural delivery position she would be forced to accept in the hospital. Also, they didn't want to expose their baby to the diseases they felt it might encounter in the hospital. In spite of these reasons, however, some of the couple's acquaintances continue to call their decision self-centered.

"I think we're more mature than that," answers the young husband. "I am thinking of the baby." Unafraid to assume the responsibility for the safety of his wife and their future child, he has a hard time understanding why most Americans totally abdicate this responsibility to the hospital.

"Who has the most to lose," he demands, "the baby or us? We have the most to lose! For the rest of our lives, if anything goes wrong, we will have to bear the burden. How can anyone insinuate we're not thinking of the baby?"[2]

His wife agrees, pointing out that 15,000 children are born each year with cerebral palsy in this country.

"I don't think of taking responsibility for yourself and your child as being illegal," she adds.

Is home birth actually illegal? That depends on who attends the birth. Having a baby at home breaks no law in itself, in the United States. In England, where medically supervised home delivery is available, do-it-yourself childbirth *is* illegal. Over here, however, the situation is reversed. A mother may legally have her baby at home with no assistance, but as soon as help arrives on the scene, the legality of home birth comes into question!

Most states have laws which regulate who may attend the birth. Although some form of midwifery is allowed in thirty-seven states, seventeen states permit only certified midwives to practice. And in two other states, if anyone besides a doctor assists at a home birth, that person may be accused of practicing medicine (or midwifery) without a license.[3]

Then what about a *licensed* midwife? More and more states are broadening their laws so that licensed midwives will be allowed to deliver babies both at home and in the hospital. California, for example, put such a bill into effect in 1975. But their law, like many, covers only certified nurse-midwives who work under the supervision of a physician.

So far, relatively few of these licensed midwives are available. A 1974 survey estimated that there were only about one hundred students per year in all present U.S. schools of nurse-midwifery.[4] As a result of this shortage, and to meet the growing demand for their presence at home births, lay midwives have begun practicing in many areas.

In March, 1974, three such midwives from the Santa Cruz, California Birth Center were arrested and charged with practicing medicine without a license. But these women deny that attending births is the same as practicing medicine. They claim that the profession of midwifery has more to do with art than with science.

"People can't understand that midwives don't deliver babies, the mother does," states one of the midwives.

"I go to assist nature as a witness to a normal event and to see that it remains normal. If it varies, we encourage people to go to a doctor or a hospital," she explains.

While the state maintains that this unusual prosecution is simply a question of licensing, supporters of the midwives view it as harassment. They also question whether it's constitutional for the state to make laws which forbid a mother to choose lay midwives and thus have the effect of forcing her to deliver in a hospital against her will. Some lawyers view the Santa Cruz case as a major battle in the war for women's liberation. At stake in the trial, they think, is women's right to control their own bodies.

"Birth is a private matter . . . not something someone else should decide for you." This opinion comes from a California mother whose son's birth was assisted by one of the Santa Cruz midwife defendants.

"Once you let the government tell a mother where she can have her baby, and who can be there, they'll start trying to tell you where and when you can have sex." Her view may sound extreme, but many share it. Like many Americans, those who want home births are jealous of their civil liberties and they resent actions which they think interfere with citizens' private lives.

Since the Santa Cruz case, a number of lay midwives in California have adopted a "hands-off" policy during home childbirth. While continuing to offer prenatal courses in nutrition and pregnancy, they attend the actual birth in a purely advisory capacity. One of the baby's parents cuts and ties the umbilical cord under the midwife's supervision. (One of the midwives points out that many of the couples she serves live in extremely remote areas and would have their babies at home whether they had professional birth attendants or not.)

Some people wonder about the parent's legal liability in the case of either the baby or mother dying during a home birth. There is no apparent history of prosecution on this point, but this does not mean that those who want a home delivery should be unaware of the possibility. In the states that prohibit all forms of midwifery, anyone besides a doctor who assists at a home birth could face manslaughter charges if a death occurs.

So the absence of precedents in certain areas doesn't mean that those who choose childbirth at home should consider themselves immune to the risk of legal action. This also applies to husbands who hope to deliver their own babies at home. Although no record could be located of a husband being prosecuted under the midwifery laws, prospective fathers should not dismiss the risk offhandedly. The California Business and Professions Code, for example, states that any person who assists at a nonemergency home birth commits a misdemeanor if he is not a doctor or a certified midwife. At the present time, this type of offense is punishable by a fine of up to $500 and/ or a term of up to six months in jail.

If complications came up and resulted in a death during this kind of home delivery, felony charges could also be brought against the unlicensed birth attendant. Once again, the fact that a state has never charged a husband under its midwifery laws does not mean that it couldn't, as long as birth attendant restrictions are on its books. (Husbands should be realistic in evaluating this risk, however. Laws prohibiting lay midwifery were made with midwives in mind, not husbands.)

Couples who think they might want to have their babies at home owe it to themselves to seek sound legal advice on all these questions. They might start by calling the state Board of Health and asking about its particular laws on home births. If the parents discover that their state restricts the attendants at home births, they should seek the advice of a lawyer.

An attorney referral service can usually be found in the yellow pages of the telephone directory. Sponsored by the local bar association, it tries to help people locate a lawyer who can best help them. If the caller requests the name of a younger attorney who might be sympathetic to the idea of childbirth at home, he will probably have better luck.

Some lawyers charge a flat fee, such as twenty-five dollars, for the initial consultation. Whatever the cost, it's worth it. Before considering home birth seriously, couples must know exactly what legal consequences surround it in their state.

The most obvious danger in a home birth, of course, centers around the possibility of either the mother or the baby developing a problem that might require immediate medical attention. Perhaps the best way to evaluate this risk is to consider the whole picture. More than nine out of ten births in our country today are considered normal. In fact, several estimates say that over 95 percent of American mothers have uncomplicated births.[5]

If a mother has a history of at least one normal birth, her chances of having another simple birth are better than 99 percent, in the opinion of one obstetrician. A group of doctors in Marin County, California, have delivered about five hundred babies since 1970, without a single maternal death. Yet almost 90 percent of their patients had their babies at home.

But supervised home childbirth has generally proved to be safer than those which take place in hospitals. Consider, for example, the records of such historic institutions as the Chicago Maternity Center. During one period years ago, the Center delivered more than 12,000 babies at home without a single maternal death. At the same time, American mothers who had their babies in hospitals died at the rate of over 2 per 1,000 births. During the 1950s, the center attended over 9,000 consecutive home births without losing a mother.[6] These statistics become doubly amazing when one learns that many of these mothers were in the "high risk" category. Often undernourished and badly housed, they frequently had large families already, and medical problems of their own as well. In fact, some experts estimate that even today, fully 80 percent of the midwife-assisted home deliveries in poverty areas are high-risk births.

High standards of safety have been set by other groups which report home deliveries. The Frontier Nursing Service, a group of midwives who attended home births in Appalachia, had no maternal mortalities for twelve years. Yet they assisted at thousands of births in the poorest of homes—houses that frequently had no indoor plumbing whatsoever. New York City's Maternity Center Association reported no maternal deaths due to postpartum bleeding during a period of twenty years. In over five thousand home deliveries, a slight percentage of the mothers suffered postpartum hemorrhages, but they were controlled at home.

"There are rare occurrences like hemorrhaging that could be aided more quickly if a woman was in a hospital," admits Allen Cohen, whose baby was born at home. But, he feels, these instances should be balanced against the risks of going to the hospital. Exposure to diseases, anesthesia deaths, childbirth drugs, and the general fear-tension-pain syndrome are only a few of these hospital-connected dangers. Furthermore, argues Cohen, the risk of unexpected childbirth-connected accidents exists no matter where the birth takes place. This risk, although minimal, is part of *every* delivery. It cannot be done away with by going to the hospital to have the baby.

"Of the twenty nations that record mortality rates in childbirth, America, where most births are in hospitals, has the second most deaths in childbirth," according to *Childbirth Is Ecstasy*.[7] Figures like this have led anthropologist Ashley Montagu to declare that in the United States, home delivery may be safer.

"My students who have had their babies at home wind up with better care than those who go to the hospital," claims Dr. Montagu.

But it is the safety of the baby which usually causes the most concern when the possibility of home birth comes up.

"There is more risk in home delivery to the infant than to the mother," asserts a California obstetrician who opposes home births. Many doctors give hospitals the credit for reducing our newborn deaths. Just during the past fifteen years, the American infant mortality rate has dropped from over 25 deaths per 1,000 births to less than 18 deaths for the same number of births. But many experts think that even this figure is too high. They point to the dozen or so other countries which have lower infant mortality rates than the United

States, yet where sizable numbers of the births still take place at home.

The problem, then, is to identify the births which will have potential problems so that they can take place in a hospital, where special equipment can be used to help make the delivery successful. It's at this point that much disagreement arises. Many doctors feel that even though only 2 percent to 4 percent of newborn infants will need intensive care, all births should occur in the hospital where such care is available. In fact, some obstetricians insist that *all* deliveries should be electronically monitored. They claim that this is the only way to detect the small number of babies who do not have problems until they are being born.

Those on the other side argue that using a fetal monitor would further mechanize a natural function. Childbirth, they assert, has been dehumanized enough in our hospitals. Instead of adding another piece of technology to find out which babies are in danger, they suggest removing those features of labor and delivery rooms which cause or contribute to dangerous deliveries.

Furthermore, about 80 percent of high-risk pregnancies can be identified in advance, according to a Sacramento, California perinatologist. (A perinatologist is a doctor who cares for sick babies before, during and after they are born.) Such a specialist can combine information from the mother's medical history with data from her prenatal checkups and predict the great majority of problem deliveries.

Women who have a history of heart disease or diabetes, for instance, run a higher risk of developing problems during pregnancy and birth. So do mothers who are over forty or still in their early teens. Women who have had difficulties with earlier deliveries, such as a breech birth, need to be closely monitored by a good obstetrician. Mothers who have a small pelvis, mothers expecting twins, mothers with anemia, fibroid tumors, liver disease, or obesity also need special care.

Since so many difficult deliveries can be recognized in

advance, prenatal care should be sought as soon as possible. Dr. George M. Ryan, Jr., chairman of the Obstetrics Practice Committee of the American College of Obstetricians and Gynecologists, advises women to see their doctors before they are ten weeks pregnant. Experts estimate that if "high-risk" women received medical care early enough in their pregnancies, prompt recognition and treatment could reduce the delivery dangers for two out of every three such mothers.[8]

Ideally, every woman should see a doctor at least six months *before* getting pregnant. She could then receive a vaccination against German measles, which causes birth defects. The vaccine should be received early, as it occasionally persists in the body for over two months. If the woman becomes pregnant during this time, the lingering effects of her immunization could affect her unborn baby.

Since the most severe birth defects are caused during the earliest days after conception, the mother may not even realize she is pregnant at the time. Informed doctors, therefore, will take steps to protect all women from damaging their unborn babies throughout their childbearing years. Any powerful drugs or X rays should be given to a fertile woman only during the two weeks immediately following menstruation to preclude the possibility of injuring her unborn infant.

"Of all pregnant women, those who plan to deliver at home need prenatal care the most," points out Michael Whitt, a doctor in a group which has assisted at several hundred home births. He agrees that one of the aims of prenatal care is to identify the small minority of high risk pregnancies. (Between 10 percent and 20 percent of Dr. Whitt's patients have their babies in hospitals—some for medical reasons and a few for personal reasons.)

Besides the women who suffer from heart, lung, or kidney diseases, or have histories which may make their next delivery risky, a very few patients develop problems *during* their pregnancies. An alert doctor will know how to interpret symptoms such as elevated blood pressure or protein in the urine. Many of these warning signs can be detected only through professional care and laboratory tests. Therefore, it's obvious that in order to be highly effective, prenatal care must begin early and be continued on a regular basis throughout pregnancy. There are simply no shortcuts in this area; skipping prenatal checkups is playing with the life of the unborn child.

Those who believe that childbirth at home is the best way to have a baby should be honest with themselves. If the mother is over thirty-two or under eighteen, if she has Rh negative blood, if she has certain diseases or a history of previous birth complications, the risks of home delivery would probably be too high. (In England, where a substantial number of births take place at home, women over thirty-five or those who live in unsuitable housing are encouraged to deliver in the hospital.)

New Miracles of Childbirth, by Elliott H. McCleary, contains a chart on page 158, which lists all the criteria commonly used to identify pregnancies that may be unusual. It's called "Are You High Risk?" This chart should be of special interest to anyone who might want to consider childbirth at home. Since it's completely objective, it could be consulted even before visiting a doctor, and it might prevent possible disappointment. If a woman discovers from the chart that she's likely to have a complicated pregnancy, at least she won't blame it on her doctor.

Home births, then, should only be considered after a physician confirms that the mother is in robust health and that the pregnancy is progressing normally. All women who are pregnant should also be on the alert for the following warning signals. These could be the first signs of possible complications. If any of them occurs, the expectant mother should call a doctor or go to a hospital.

—— Severe, persistent abdominal pain
—— Vaginal bleeding

—— Dim or blurry vision
—— Swelling of the face, eyes or fingers
—— Chills or fever
—— Severe headache during the last three months
—— Absence of daily fetal movement after the fifth
month

Hopefully, very few parents would allow themselves to become so alienated by hospital technocracy that they would refuse to go to one during a clear-cut medical emergency. People who work in the home delivery field warn parents not to close their minds against hospitals completely.

In 1974, a California woman, a registered nurse who worked in a Berkeley hospital until the birth of her first baby, was counting on having it at home. She changed her mind, however, when her labor lasted more than twenty hours.

"I'm really glad that the hospital was there and that I could go there for help when I needed it," she admitted. Confessing that she had felt extreme disappointment about having to go to the hospital, she thinks other parents could learn from her experience.

"It would be better to plan and hope to have your baby at home, but realize that there is also the possibility of going to the hospital. So you should plan for that, too."

Couples who opt for home delivery should do everything they can to insure that the birth of their baby will go smoothly. They can take comfort in the fact that over 95 percent of prepared births are normal. Yet they must face the possibility that they may be among the 5 percent who will encounter problems during the delivery.

Some doctors frequently seem quick to exaggerate this possibility.

"To the patient who has a successful home delivery, it's all an especially meaningful, almost mystical experience. To the one who loses her baby, it's a tragedy." This warning comes from Dr. Phillip Goldstein, chief obstetrician at San Francisco General Hospital.

Conscientious parents may then wonder whether they have a moral obligation to have their baby in a hospital, in case it needs immediate attention that can only be provided there. Some resolve this doubt by turning to guidelines from various religious faiths. According to the teaching of the Catholic Church, for example, it would be wrong to fail to supply the ordinary means for preserving life. But neither the parent nor the physician has any obligation to use *extraordinary* means to preserve life. Because of this standard, Catholic parents may feel that they must help a newborn baby to breathe by simple resuscitative methods, but they are not obliged to subject their stillborn infant to drastic emergency surgery.

"After all," argues a mother who holds this conviction, "God is the ultimate author of life and death. You get to a point where you have to make the best decision and leave the rest in God's hands."

A priest who is an expert on moral questions agrees with this. Childbirth at home, he says, is completely permissible as long as there are no medical indications against it. On the other hand, if an obstetrician has good reason to fear the birth may be complicated, the mother has a moral obligation to deliver in the hospital if it's at all possible for her to do so. This advice coincides with the view expressed in *The Experience of Childbirth,* by Sheila Kitzinger. Mrs. Kitzinger, a distinguished British childbirth educator and social anthropologist, offers this opinion:

> Unless there are reasons why it is best for the baby to be born in the hospital (either medical or 'social' reasons, which include not having sufficient room), home is . . . the best place to have the baby, but, of course, in those cases where difficulties are likely to crop up the hospital is by far the safer place to be.

Parents should realize, too, that there are a certain number of stillbirths which are unavoidable. Even doctors who strongly oppose home delivery admit that there is a "hard core of fetal deaths which will occur regardless of where delivery takes place."[9] People who can accept this fact will probably realize that if their baby turns out to be in this group, the loss may be far more bearable if the birth takes place at home.

Although the specter of a stillborn baby haunts most parents-to-be, the possibility must be faced whether the birth takes place at home or in the hospital. Even the most modern perinatal center cannot magically instill life into a baby who is born dead. Some people think that parents who have their children at home are better prepared for this outcome, since they accept the responsibility from the outset. In *Birth Book,* midwife Raven Lang writes about a mother who gives birth to a stillborn baby.

> She feels her birth was beautiful and natural. Great sorrow is felt in the death but also a great acceptance. There was not the usual response to death from anyone of us. There was birth—there was death, all at once.

Some psychologists think that the loss of stillbirth would be easier for the *other children* in the family as well, if it follows a home delivery.

"If the birth is not successful, the shared experience of the loss is the more readily understood, as he is supported by those he trusts," says one California mother.

Many thoughtful sociologists recognize the emotional damage caused by our lack of exposure to both birth and death. In our culture, removing these natural events to the antiseptic confines of the hospital has resulted in an unnatural fear of both. When birth and death occur in the home, however, acceptance and understanding can replace the unnatural dread most Americans now evince toward both the beginning and end of life.

Some people say that losing a newborn infant is bad enough, but losing a baby amidst the technology of an infant intensive care unit can push even the most stoic parents to the emotional breaking point. Anyone can surely sympathize with the parents of multiple-birth premature babies as they spend anxious weeks surrounded by respirators, intravenous equipment, and bulletins on the deteriorating conditions of their tiny two-pound infants.

If an infant death takes place at a home birth, the atmosphere is very different. In *birth*, by Caterine Milinaire, the story is told of a young woman who had a stillborn baby at home. Despite the presence of a doctor, the baby's heartbeat gradually grew fainter as labor progressed, and she was born dead. Suffering from grief and shock, the mother was still glad she'd had the baby at home.

> Anyway, it was easier to have this trip go down in a home, rather than in a hospital. I was surrounded by people who loved me, who cried with me and who didn't make me feel ashamed over so much emotion. I wasn't shut away in a sterile little room with a perfect view of beaming new mothers, their arms and breasts filled with babies while I lay all empty, aching, titties abrim with surplus milk.[11]

When a young California couple lost their first baby during its unassisted home birth, they buried it together near their mountain home.

"These people are understanding when that happens and if it happens again, they'll bury it in the woods again," said the male midwife who attended the birth of their next child. Fortunately, the tragedy did not repeat itself. Their second baby was born uneventfully in 1974. (When a lawyer heard about their first stillborn baby, he warned other parents that burying a body anywhere besides a cemetery might be against the law in some jurisdictions.)

This couple's experience illustrates the advantage of having outside help for childbirth at home. If the delivery turns out to be among the 5 percent or so which have problems, the presence of a doctor or midwife can dramatically increase the odds of having a successful birth. A competent attendant, then, can be viewed as a sort of insurance policy. Outside assistance at a home delivery helps protect the couple against that slight chance that something may go wrong. Naturally, the parents expect and hope they won't need this protection. But it's better to have this insurance than to put all their faith in statistics.

When all the legal and medical risks are considered, it becomes obvious that home delivery is not for everyone. Whoever thinks that they might want to have a baby at home ought to first place themselves in the care of a competent doctor. Second, they should seek advice from a good attorney so they can understand what their legal risks might be. Only after they fully understand both their medical and legal options will they be able to make an informed decision about childbirth at home.

Even if a couple believes they're in the clear medically and legally, they should scrutinize their own deep-seated attitudes toward home delivery. People who really think the hospital is the safest place to have their baby would no doubt feel uncomfortable with a home birth. One midwife tells the story of a young couple who asked her to attend the birth of their first child. As her labor progressed, however, the midwife realized the girl felt frightened.

"It turned out she was a doctor's daughter," reports the midwife. "She trusted doctors and was comfortable in hospitals. When she went into labor, she instinctively wanted to go to a hospital."

As soon as the midwife realized this, she called an ambulance and took the girl to the nearest hospital for the birth.

Unfortunately, some mothers-to-be opt for childbirth at home because of peer pressure. In a few communities, home delivery has become something of a fad. This seems to be especially common among people who espouse alternate and radical life-styles. A couple living in a communal type of arrangement may think they must have a home birth because it's expected of them. Doctors and midwives who attend these deliveries often express concern about this attitude. They think the people may have chosen to have their babies at home for the wrong reasons.

Deciding to have a baby at home takes time. Many factors should be taken into consideration, and many ingrained attitudes must be closely examined. Nature wisely allots the parents several months to plan and prepare for their baby's birth; it would not be foolish to use much of this time thinking about where the birth might best take place.

Some couples approach the decision one step at a time. During the early part of pregnancy, they search for a good doctor and find out what types of delivery are available in local maternity wards. They read up on various birth methods.

As the pregnancy progresses, home birth could become a more vital issue. Whether or not a couple pursues any alternative birth style depends on many factors. If only conventional delivery is available in their community, and the couple has strong reservations about its safety, they will probably investigate the possibility of home delivery more actively. Hopefully, they will obtain legal advice before committing themselves. And hopefully, they won't become so set on a home birth that they would refuse hospital care during an emergency.

They should also feel sure they won't worry about what other people will say, no matter how the birth turns out.

Finally, the parents may decide to look for a doctor or midwife who would be willing to come to their house for the birth. For many people, the decision to have their baby at home may rest upon the quality of help they are able to locate.

Who should attend childbirth at home? How can parents find reliable assistance during labor and delivery? These questions will be discussed in the next chapter.

NOTES

1. Lester Dessez Hazell, *Commonsense Childbirth* (New York: G.P. Putnam's Sons, 1969), p. 142.
2. Hilary Abramson, "Why Can't Mothers Deliver Their Babies at Home?" *The Sacramento Union*, May 5, 1974, p. E8.
3. Kaye Yost, "At Home Or In The Hospital?" *California Living* Sunday magazine of *San Francisco Examiner*), November 3, 1974, p. 11. Also Elliott H. McCleary, *New Miracles of Childbirth*, (New York: David McKay Co., 1974), p. 212.
4. Elizabeth B. Connell, M.D., "The Modern Nurse-Midwife," *Redbook*, July 1974, p. 66.
5. "What You Should Know About Having a Baby at Home," *Glamour*, March 1974, p. 39.
6. Helen Wessell, *Natural Childbirth and the Family* (New York: Harper & Row), 1973, p. 240.
7. Allen Cohen, *Childbirth Is Ecstasy* (San Francisco: Aquarius, 1971), p. 72.
8. "How Pregnancy Dangers Are Being Reduced," *Good Housekeeping*, January 1974, p. 124.
9. Kaye Yost, op. cit., p. 6.
10. "What the Readers Think (Childbirth)," *California Living*, December 8, 1974, p. 60.
11. Caterine Milinaire, *birth* (New York: Harmony Books, 1974), p. 161.

OTHER SOURCES
(listed as they appear in text)

Linda Kramer, "Childbirth at Home," *The Sacramento Union*, October 27, 1974, p. C6.

Veronica Meidus, "Three Midwives Called Criminals; Attorney Cries 'Unconstitutional'," *The California Libertarian News*, July 4, 1974, p. 2.

Interview with Michael Whitt, M.D., Point Reyes, California, May 10, 1974.

Department of Obstetrics and Gynecology, "Information For Maternity Patients," USAF Hospital, Maxwell AFB, Alabama.

Susan Eisenhower Bradshaw, "Two Jam Jars, One Bucket, Two Pudding Basins" (Home Birth, a Personal Account), *The Saturday Evening Post*, May 1974, p. 75.

Russell Shaw, "Controversy over Euthanasia," *The Catholic Free Press*, June 2, 1972.

Sheila Kitzinger, *The Experience of Childbirth* (New York: Taplinger Publishing Company, 1962.)

Raven Lang, *Birth Book* (Ben Lomond, California: Genesis Press, 1972).

Interview with Three Midwives, Santa Rosa, California, December 11, 1973.

6

BIRTH ATTENDANTS

If you were an expectant mother in primitive times, your husband would be the one to help you when your baby was born. In *Awake and Aware,* Dr. Irwin Chabon states that birth attendance was introduced into human culture very early, with husbands as the first probable assistants. Since primitive peoples lived in small family units quite a distance apart from each other, it must have seemed only natural for the male to help his mate during labor and delivery.

It's believed that, besides offering the woman companionship and comfort in her travail, the husband sat behind his wife, supporting her and pressing on her abdomen when she had contractions. No doubt he also cut and tied the cord, wiping and swaddling the newborn baby afterwards.

While thousands of years of civilization have changed many aspects of the human condition, the simple physiology of birth has remained the same. Eve gave birth to Cain and Abel by a process that was biologically identical to the way the most modern mother has her baby today. Of course, poor Eve didn't receive any of the pain-relieving drugs an American mother gets, but Adam's presence in the delivery room probably helped to compensate!

Like Adam and Eve, many couples today take a down-to-earth attitude about the way they have their children. Often feeling resentful about the way the government seems to either tax or license everything they do, such couples believe that their right to arrange the circumstances of their deliveries equals their right to decide their own wedding arrangements. Bill Holmes, a young man in Berkeley, California, typifies this independent stance:

"There's no reason to depend on the capitalistic system if you can do something outside it and can do it in a more relaxed and friendly, open way," says Bill. "Having a baby at home fits in with our whole life-style."

Bill also appreciated the experience of home birth because he was able to actively participate in it. He cut the umbilical cord that connected the baby to his wife, Annie. Although Bill helped during the birth, a midwife and pediatrician were present, too. They were equipped with a fetus-cope, suction apparatus, clamps for the cord, sterile gloves, eyedrops for the baby, and medicine to control bleeding in the mother. In fact, some people would say that the Holmes's delivery received better care at home than it would have received in many hospitals.

Who should attend childbirth at home? Or should anyone have her baby by herself? Although most women are glad to have assistance at this time, a few do not welcome it. One such lady, Mrs. Patricia C. Carter, is practically in a class by herself. After having her first baby lamed by a forceps delivery, and her second baby held back by force and later given to another woman in the hospital by mistake, she had her next seven children at home. She did not even allow her husband, an Army brigadier general, to help her. A newspaper reporter who took pictures of the birth of Mrs. Carter's last baby in 1956 confirmed that she handled the birth with ease, dignity, and finesse.

In 1957, Mrs. Carter published *Come Gently, Sweet Lucina;* her book can be regarded as something of a collector's item, being the first do-it-yourself manual on home birth to appear in this country. To be sure, other books give instructions on how to attend deliveries, but these are usually written by doctors for medical students, midwives, or policemen. Mrs. Carter's book is written by a mother and tells women how to deliver their own babies.

Mrs. Carter founded the League of Liberated Women in 1959. It awards its members certificates of emancipation which say:

> Because she chose to, and did, bear a child . . . without the attendance of physician, nurse, or midwife, which evidences liberation from the false belief now generally prevalent in our Time and Society, namely that the presence of a professional birth attendant is necessary or desirable even in cases where no mental or emotional disease is present in the mother, and where no physical disease or deformity exists in mother or child, and where no malpresentation or malproportion exists, . . . we hereby award her LIFETIME MEMBERSHIP in THE LEAGUE OF LIBERATED WOMEN.

Few American women, however, are as resourceful as Mrs. Carter. Although most mothers could give birth alone if they had to, (and in many parts of the world they still do) a birth attendant is a big help. Besides caring for the newborn infant immediately, an attendant can provide reassurance to the woman as her contractions grow stronger. As the pace of labor increases, many women become apprehensive and wonder if they are going to make it through the delivery. They should have someone with them constantly, preferably someone they are close to emotionally.

"The sick lie in coma surrounded by loved ones, while the healthy in labor lie alone," writes Dr. Chabon in *Awake and Aware*. Unfortunately, this is how most labors are conducted in our hospitals. Usually, there are not enough nurses to stay with a laboring woman, and if there is more than one mother in the labor room, their husbands may not be allowed to stay with them, either.

Mothers who have had their babies at home usually say that one of the best things about it was having constant company while they were in labor. Unlike being in the hospital, they didn't have to worry about being separated from their husbands. Furthermore, many women appreciate the opportunity to have their babies in privacy. Lying on her own bed, amidst familiar surroundings and the people who love her, the mother's relaxation may be so complete that the birth feels relatively painless.

If having babies at home is so easy, why bother with an outside birth attendant? Wouldn't the husband be good enough? For most births, the answer is yes. In more than nine out of ten cases, the delivery will take place normally no matter what anyone does or doesn't do. But in the tenth birth, if a sudden problem crops up, an experienced birth attendant can make a difference that is truly vital.

Most Americans of childbearing age today expect a doctor to deliver their babies. Yet men as birth attendants are relative newcomers. Except for a few priests and male physicians in ancient Egypt and Greece, the traditional birth attendant has been the midwife. Not until the use of forceps by the Chamberlain brothers in the sixteenth century did male physicians and surgeons reenter the childbirth field.

"It is of great significance that the attendance of male midwives followed closely upon the introduction of forceps into childbirth," writes midwife Raven Lang in her *Birth Book*. As the centuries passed and further scientific inventions were introduced into obstetrics, the interest of male doctors increased.

"When every woman realizes and every physician insists that childbearing deserves the same consideration as a major surgical operation, then and then only will a woman reap the greatest benefits from anesthesia," stated one doctor in 1920. Perhaps we should not blame obstetricians for feeling this way, since obstetrics-gynecology is considered a branch of surgery.

More American women probably ought to ponder this point. According to obstetrician Jack Schneider, one of the directors of the University of Wisconsin's perinatal center, a doctor's interest in obstetrics is more important than what kind of degree he has on his office wall. Just because a given doctor is a FACOG (Fellow, American College of Obstetricians and Gynecologists) doesn't mean that he likes to deliver babies. His special training may be in surgery, with a subspecialty in gynecology.[1]

What many couples consider an ideal birth attendant today, however, is not a white-coated professional who will deliver their baby, but rather a sympathetic assistant who will be ready to use his medical training should it be needed. One of the reasons for the rapidly growing popularity of home childbirth, in fact, is that women are realizing that a lack of "professionalism" is often an advantage when it comes to receiving humane care.[2]

"Ideally, the obstetrician's role is to stand by. He is there—like an insurance policy—in case anything goes wrong," says Dr. H.M.I. Liley in *Pregnancy, Childbirth and the Newborn Baby.*

Unfortunately, only a minuscule number of American doctors see this as their role during the labors and deliveries of their women patients. But another group of childbirth experts does—midwives. As they have done traditionally, midwives deliver about 80 percent of the babies born in the world today. In fact, midwives were still delivering almost half of the the babies born in New York City as recently as 1905. And in every country that has a lower infant mortality rate than the United States, nurse-midwives are the predominant birth attendants.[3]

> Professional midwives handle the majority of normal births in such technologically advanced countries as Sweden, Germany, and the Netherlands. In England, which

has one of the world's most advanced health-care systems, 80 percent of all births are handled by midwives.[4]

Wherever midwives have been used in the United States,
too, they have significantly lowered the infant death rate. In
1970, Holmes County, Mississippi lost only 17 babies for every
1,000 births. In 1969, before five nurse-midwives arrived, the
neonatal death rate in the county was 39 per 1,000.[5]

Besides improving the infant death rate, midwives usually achieve a lowering of maternal deaths. When the Frontier
Nursing Service sent nurse-midwives into Appalachia almost
fifty years ago, their first 10,000 deliveries had a maternal
death rate of only one per 1,000. (The maternal mortality rate
for the whole country at the time was three times higher.)[6] In
the past twenty years, the Frontier Nursing Service has not
lost a single mother during childbirth.

There are several different kinds of midwives. Besides
the nurse-midwife, whose "new" role in American medicine
has been much publicized recently, we presently keep three
other groups busy: lay midwives, granny midwives, and professional midwives from foreign countries.

Of the four categories, granny midwives have been
around the longest. These old-fashioned "granny women"
delivered the majority of Americans at home until around the
1930s. Their records seem to be quite good, considering the
fact that they learned by experience and had little or no
medical training. And if they got paid cash at all, it was usually
only two or three dollars for each birth.

"Aunt Lizzie" Keason, who lived in Tiger, Georgia, was
one of its best-known and well-loved midwives. This is how
she described her craft.

> Many's the time I left home before daylight and returned
> after dark. I remember bringing 9 children into the
> world for one couple. I walked through snow and ice
> —more than two miles . . . I didn't lose a single mother
> or baby in those more than 525 times. I thank God for
> that.[7]

In 1943, when the area where Aunt Lizzie worked opened one of the first maternity centers in the rural South, the granny midwives were able to receive formal training and upgrade their skills. At the center, they learned about anatomy, nutrition, prenatal care, and sterile technique. Even more important, they were taught noninterference; midwives were to avoid performing vaginal examinations, and they were to call in the doctor promptly if their clients showed symptoms of abnormal labor.

According to the midwives interviewed in *Foxfire 2*, birth-connected deaths were very infrequent. Like "Aunt Lizzie" Keason, many midwives assisted at hundreds of births without a single maternal or infant death. Perhaps for this reason, they believed that the mothers who had home deliveries fared better than those who went to hospitals.

"You hardly ever heared of one a' dyin', and you very seldom heared of one a' bein' deformed in any way," reported one of the grannies. "Most of 'em had big families then," she continued. "And they done better at home than they do these that went and had they'rn at th' hospital."[8]

Granny midwives delivered about 33,000 American babies in 1968, mostly in the South. (The majority of them earned between ten and twenty-five dollars for each birth.) Although there are some grannies who are still practicing, most of them have been legislated out of existence. According to one source, doctors first launched a massive propaganda campaign against midwives around 1900. In order to persuade women to deliver in the hospital, obstetricians would describe the midwives as "filthy whores with grimy fingers."[9] Once such seeds of mistrust had been planted, mothers began to avoid calling midwives.

But the doctors' motives may not have been completely selfish. Upset by our high maternal and infant mortality rates, many obstetricians thought that if they could convince all women to have their babies in the hospital, the problem would be solved. To the doctors, of course, midwives were part of the problem. Their "ignorance" and lack of sterile technique were thought to be responsible for our high national birth-connected death rate.[10] (Many doctors still believe that the increased use of hospitals for births will lower our maternal and infant death rates, apparently unaware of the fact that midwives and home births in many other countries produce fewer infant mortalities.)

For the most part, granny midwives in America have gone the way of the horse and buggy. A 1973 article in *Ms.*, however, estimated that there are still about five thousand grannies today in such diverse places as Appalachia, Mississippi, the Texas border and coastal California.

But this article included *all* American lay midwives. Usually the younger women, such as those who serve California's counterculture, are distinguished from the old-fashioned granny midwives. Unlike the granny women, the young lay midwife today may have much more formal education. Some have had nurse's training. A well-known Santa Rosa, California midwife has a degree in public health. Several other midwives are married to doctors.

Lay midwives often make up in experience what they lack in formal preparation. Doctors or midwives may allow interested women to accompany them when they attend home births. The young women are then considered apprentice midwives. Gradually, the apprentices take more and more responsibility for the deliveries, until they are ready to do them on their own.

Lay midwives, however, do not "deliver" babies; they "catch" them instead. They believe the word "deliver" connotes the image of a doctor cutting open a patient's perineum and dragging out her baby. Lay midwives don't perform any such obstetrical maneuvers. This is why they maintain that the state has no right to accuse them of practicing medicine without a license. While obstetrics may well be considered a science, midwives consider their profession an art.

"If you stand around and offer a woman advice while she's giving birth, is that treatment?" questions Dr. Sheldon

Greenfield, a member of UCLA's paramedics school. "Not in a medical sense."

Several other professionals in the fields of medicine and law share this view. To them, the 1974 arrest of three midwives in Santa Cruz, California, raises the whole question of why we consider childbirth an event requiring medical attention.

"You know, there's nothing magical about men going to medical school and learning where the vagina is and how the baby comes out," states lawyer Charles Garry.[11]

The State Board of Medical Examiners apparently feels differently. Claiming that they act on "complaints from individuals who have been treated by lay midwives," they periodically investigate their activities. In Santa Cruz, armed state investigators lured two midwives to a fake birth and arrested a third midwife at the local Birth Center where her prenatal class was admiring a two-week-old baby.

Such heavy-handed tactics were greatly resented by the local community; many of its young children are among the 300 born at home in the presence of the accused midwives. As a result, hundreds of vocal supporters attended every appearance of the midwives at the county courthouse in Santa Cruz.

"We really appreciate the unbelievable community support we've had here and nationally," said Mrs. Jeannine Walker, a defendant who is the wife of a local doctor.

Perhaps another reason these three midwives have attracted national attention has been their excellent safety record. In over three hundred home births, they have had no maternal or infant deaths during childbirth.

Lay midwives in other areas of California have attended several hundred births with equally good results or with just one or two stillborn infants. One of the reasons for this success lies in their conservative handling of births—("baby-catching" rather than "delivering"). Another reason is that when a midwife suspects that a birth may become complicated, she takes the woman to a hospital as soon as possible. Some birth centers, in fact, have sent as many as 25 percent of their mothers to doctors and hospitals for specialized care.

"We're very responsible when it comes to complications," a midwife affirms. "One doctor told us he feels very safe about the Birth Center because we get scared easily. If something starts happening that anyone feels is out of the ordinary, we're off to the hospital."[12]

If lay midwives provide such conscientious care, why don't doctors accept them and recognize them as professionals? Most often, doctors cite the lay midwives' lack of formal training as the reason. People who disagree say that doctors often guard their prerogatives jealously. They may be reluctant to admit that an unlicensed midwife can help mothers deliver healthy babies as well as a doctor can. And as long as lay midwives remain unlicensed, their legal problems will probably continue to keep them "underground" in states which restrict birth attendants.

"I'd love to have a license and do this all legally and aboveboard," says one of the arrested Santa Cruz midwives. "But we're not the people that the medical establishment wants at all."

What type of midwives *are* acceptable to doctors? Apparently, only nurses who can be educated, licensed, and controlled. In 1970, the American College of Obstetricians and Gynecologists, in conjunction with the American College of Nurse-Midwives, extended formal recognition to licensed midwives.

"Qualified nurse-midwives, when working with a physician, may assume responsibility for the complete care of uncomplicated maternity patients," stated the president of the ACOG.[13] A "qualified" midwife, then, is a graduate nurse, a R.N. who has received a degree in midwifery after an extra year of training in obstetrics and gynecology. If, in addition, she takes a year of internship, she will receive a master's degree along with her nurse-midwifery certificate.

The maternity care provided by nurse-midwives is of unusually high quality. In fact, increasing numbers of doctors say that for normal deliveries, midwives provide *better* care than doctors.

"Because they are women, I believe they understand women better," says a young obstetrics resident in the Bronx. "A busy obstetrician might induce labor or use a forceps just to save time. But if the patient has a trained midwife, this couldn't happen."[14]

Another doctor, who is in charge of the obstetrics service at Roosevelt Hospital in New York, agrees that the maternity patients who have midwives have a better chance of delivering a healthy undamaged baby. His reasons? Midwives do not rush the mothers through the deliveries, and they tend to give fewer harmful drugs. Less medication given to the mother, says another doctor, means less chance of a forceps delivery. And fewer forceps deliveries leads to increased safety for unborn babies.

One of the reasons nurse-midwives don't use drugs as much as doctors is that they remain with the mother constantly. Often, the midwife meets the couple at the door of the hospital and stays with them until after the birth is over. Mothers who had midwives attend their births appreciated their continuing presence more than any other aspect of their care. All the mothers preferred it to the periodic checks they had received from their busy obstetricians during previous labors.

Usually, the midwife is able to help the mother relax so well that she can handle her labor pains with little or no pain-relieving drugs. According to many experts, "the reassurance a nurse-midwife can provide during labor is more priceless than any medication."[15]

Mothers agree. According to them, the midwife is often the one person who makes her labor bearable.

"Sandra was there to explain what was happening during the whole six hours of labor. She gave me confidence that I was going to come through it all right," testifies one mother.

"She thinks of all the little things doctors don't have time to talk about," says another woman.

Nurse-midwives have also introduced some humanizing innovations to maternity wards. In their efforts to make the hospital as homelike as possible, they have pushed for such changes as husbands in the delivery room, the "propped" position on the delivery table, and immediate breast-feeding after birth. In several hospitals, midwives have performed so many "miracles" that the maternity wards seem virtually transformed.

As a group, there are only two drawbacks to nurse-midwives. First, besides a few rare exceptions like the Frontier Nursing Service in Appalachia, most nurse-midwives assist only at hospital births. The typical nurse-midwife considers herself very much a part of an obstetrical team. Also, the legislation which permits her to deliver babies usually specifies that she must work under the supervision of a doctor. Even if a state does not restrict nurse-midwives, they may be afraid to assist at home births without malpractice insurance, which many cannot afford.

The other drawback is the relative scarcity of nurse-midwives. There are fewer than 1,500 certified midwives in the United States today. Furthermore, of the 117 programs for training obstetrical assistants, only 16 are for nurse-midwives.[16] The rest train nurse-practitioners, nurse-clinicians, and nurse-specialists—none of whom actually deliver babies.

There exists yet another group of midwives in this country. They are the more than 1,200 professional midwives from foreign countries. Most of them have graduated from schools of midwifery in England, Scotland, Ireland, Wales or Australia. With experience gained from both home and hospital deliveries in their native countries, these midwives sometimes have delivered thousands of babies by the time they are in their mid-thirties. Maybe this helps to explain why some experienced observers in this field say they perform better than most American doctors.

Even American-trained midwives receive more training in obstetrics than does the average doctor because the education of midwives usually centers around pregnancy and childbirth, whereas it's only a small part of the average medical school program. (In an increasing number of medical schools, obstetrics is no longer even a required course.)[17] Also, fewer medical students are specializing in obstetrics. By 1970, about 15 percent of the residencies in obstetrics stood vacant; of those which were filled, one-third were occupied by graduates of foreign medical schools, according to an American College of Obstetricians and Gynecologists' newsletter.

On the outside, things are about the same, and the general practitioners are not meeting the demand for birth assistants, either. In fact, according to an article in *Saturday Review of Science,* each year fewer general practitioners are doing obstetrics.

At the present time, then, we have a curious paradox. With fewer doctors delivering babies, and fewer medical students even learning how to deliver babies, the demand for midwives has never been higher. Yet the dozen-odd midwife-training programs in our country graduate only slightly over a hundred certified midwives per year.

Perhaps such obvious inequalities between supply and demand help to explain why the number of lay midwives has increased so rapidly just since 1970. The Northern California Association of Midwives, for example, has about thirty active members. By 1974, they had "caught" over five hundred babies at home, and each year they help more couples.

How does a couple find a midwife who would be willing to assist at a home birth? Either by moving to an area that has a home birth center, such as Berkeley, California, or by searching long and hard. Since lay midwives are illegal in many states, they do not advertise! Frequently, however, a midwife can be located if the couple tries hard enough. Sometimes the

State Department of Health will be willing to say which counties have lay midwives. Other times, doctors or nurses can steer people in the right direction. More than one obstetrician who only does hospital deliveries allows his nurse to go to the patients who insist on having their babies at home.

Women who are pregnant or have babies may know where to find a midwife, especially if they look "hip." Also, inquiring at food co-ops or health food stores sometimes turns up some information on the home birth scene. People who work in community or underground newspaper offices, "hip" bookstores, poster shops or even boutiques may turn out to have the necessary leads on locating a midwife.

If couples fail to find a local midwife, what should they do? There are many options still open to them, but their next step might well depend on what section of the country they live in. If there is a midwife available in a neighboring state, for example, and she lives less than two hours away by car, she might be willing to come for the birth.

Mothers who live on the West Coast may be more successful in locating help for a home birth since lay midwives practice from Vancouver, British Columbia to San Diego, California.

Couples who live on the East Coast, however, will no doubt have a much more difficult time finding a midwife. They might get better results by investigating the possibility of a home birth with another type of attendant. One approach might be to pick a local doctor who is really interested in natural childbirth, go to him for prenatal care, and hope that he will modify his views on childbirth at home as he gets to know you.

"An increasing number of private physicians scattered around the country are willing to perform home deliveries," reports a 1972 article in *Life*. There are even a few organizations which routinely send doctors into homes to attend births. The Chicago Maternity Center, for example, provides physicians and medical students for home deliveries from Northwestern University's McGaw Medical Center.

A few couples have managed to impress their obstetricians with their logical arguments in favor of childbirth at home. Once in a while, a sympathetic doctor will take the attitude that while he would be unwilling to participate in a planned home delivery, the couple should call him in case of complications. Or he may provide some other qualified form of assistance, such as the name of a nurse who works in the delivery room.

When we had our fifth baby, an obstetrical nurse came to the house after the birth to make sure that everything was all right. While this is admittedly not the safest variation of childbirth at home, it's much better than no assistance at all. A nurse with maternity ward experience can confirm that the baby is in good shape, and she can tell whether the mother needs medication to help prevent too much bleeding.*

If a couple wants a home delivery, and they are unable to locate any help whatsoever, should they still go ahead with it? This decision is one that each couple must make for itself. Increasing numbers of young people, however, are going to physicians for prenatal care, seeking reassurance that their pregnancies are progressing normally, and then going on to have their babies at home.

Is this fair to the doctor? In some areas of the United States, this is the only way that a mother who plans on home delivery can get prenatal care. If a woman tells her physician at the outset that she wants to have a home birth, most often the doctor will not accept her as a patient. Very, very few obstetricians will even consent to talk to a pregnant woman who plans to have her baby at home.

---

* Postnatal visits by nurse-midwives may also be provided by the Maternal Care Unit of a city's Visiting Nurses Association. To find out whether your area is served by a VNA, look in the yellow pages of the telephone directory under "Nurses."

According to *Birth Book,* the Santa Cruz Birth Center got started as a direct result of the local doctors' refusal to see such patients. Midwife Raven Lang writes: "No O.B. in town would give prenatal care to women who planned to deliver at home."

Yet doctors who attend both home and hospital deliveries insist that women who want home births need scrupulous prenatal care. And they view their colleagues' refusal to supply it as "ethically indefensible."

"In my opinion, any M.D. who refuses to see these girls is, ipso facto, guilty of malpractice," states Dr. Michael Whitt, a general practitioner in Point Reyes Station, California.

The overwhelming majority of obstetricians, however, remain adamantly opposed to childbirth at home and unwilling to supply prenatal care to a home delivery patient. Yet, somehow, the woman who plans to have her baby at home must obtain medical supervision during her pregnancy. How to get it is explained in the next chapter.

NOTES

1. Elliott H. McCleary, *New Miracles of Childbirth* (New York: David McKay Company, 1974), p. 148.
2. Ellen Frankfort, *Vaginal Politics* (New York: Quadrangle Books, 1972), p. 91.
3. Judy Klemesrud, "Why Women Are Losing Faith in Their Doctors," *McCalls,* June 1973, p. 122.
4. "Return of the Midwife," *Time,* November 20, 1972, p. 56.
5. Patrick Young, "The Throughly Modern Midwife," *Saturday Review of Science,* September 2, 1972, p. 42.
6. Elizabeth B. Connell, M.D., "The Modern Nurse-Midwife," *Redbook,* July 1974, p. 64.
7. Eliot Wigginton, ed., *Foxfire 2* (Garden City, New York: Anchor Press/Doubleday, 1973), p. 283.
8. Ibid, p. 293.
9. Ellen Frankfort, op. cit., p. 89.
10. Shirley Streshinsky, "Are You Safer With a Midwife?" *Ms.,* October 1973, p. 26.

11. David Talbott and Barbara Zheutlin, "The Legalities of Attending a Birth," *Rolling Stone,* May 23, 1974, p. 12.
12. Ibid.
13. Patrick Young, op. cit., p. 43.
14. Marian Behan Hammer, "The Midwife: A New Image," *Marriage,* December 1973, p. 24.
15. Nancy Axelrod Comer, "Midwifery: Would You Let This Woman Deliver Your Child?" *Mademoiselle,* June 1973, p. 182.
16. Elliott H. McCleary, op. cit., p. 207.
17. Ellen Frankfort, op. cit., p. 90.

OTHER SOURCES
(listed as they appear in the text)

Irwin Chabon, *Awake and Aware* (New York: Delacorte Press, 1966.)
Linda Kramer, "Childbirth at Home," *The Sacramento Union,* October 27, 1974, p. C6.
Patricia C. Carter, *Come Gently, Sweet Lucina* (Titusville, Florida: Patricia Cloyd Carter, 1957.)
Raven Lang, *Birth Book* (Ben Lomond, California: Genesis Press, 1972.)
H.M.I. Liley, M.D., and Beth Day, *Pregnancy, Childbirth and the Newborn Baby* (New York: Random House, 1967.)
Marj Von B, "Accused Santa Cruz Midwives Rally Defenders," *Watsonville (Calif.) Register-Pajaronian,* March 26, 1974.
Dorothea M. Lang, "The Midwife Returns—Modern Style," *Parents,* October 1972.
Interview with Three Midwives, Santa Rosa, California, December 11, 1973.
G. Breu, ed., "Birth on the Kitchen Table," *Life,* August 18, 1972, p. 54.
Interview with Dr. Michael Whitt, Point Reyes, California, May 10, 1974.

7

HOW TO PREPARE FOR
CHILDBIRTH AT HOME

If you want to have a healthy baby, get prenatal care several months before you're pregnant! This may sound like putting the cart before the horse, but if the mother takes care of certain things *before* conception, her pregnancy will be easier for her and less hazardous for her baby.

Many doctors advise young women to have a complete physical checkup six months before they get married. An internal pelvic examination is also recommended, since as many as 10 percent of brides-to-be suffer from simple vaginal infections.[1] (Most of these can be cleared up quite simply with antibiotics, but they are easier to treat if the woman is not pregnant.) During a pelvic exam, a gynecologist can also identify any conditions which might make pregnancy extra hazardous, such as fibroid tumors.

This prepregnancy checkup is also a good time for women to be innoculated with measles-mumps-rubella vaccine, if they haven't had these diseases in childhood. The rubella innoculation should be taken several months before pregnancy, to avoid exposing the embryo to German measles.

Also, to protect the developing baby during the early

130

weeks of pregnancy, all other medicines should be avoided. Antibiotics like tetracycline can cause fetal damage, and cortisone preparations are suspected of causing harmful alterations. Some antihistamines cause malformed infants, as do two of the most commonly prescribed tranquilizers.[2] If a mother is addicted to heroin, morphine, Demerol or methadone during pregnancy, her baby will suffer from withdrawal symptoms which will make him very sick and may even kill him.[3]

> A major difficulty in preventing birth defects caused by drugs is the fact that these substances do most of their damage in the earliest weeks after conception. The infant's body, including brain and heart, have already begun to form before his mother has missed her first menstrual period . . . By the time most women have the first appointment with a physician to confirm the pregnancy, much of the danger of major malformations has passed and the physicians's warning about the hazards of drugs and chemicals comes too late to prevent much possible damage.[4]

When a woman has a prepregnancy checkup, the doctor may allow her to get a chest X ray; since X rays can cause damage to the unborn child, it makes sense to have even a chest X ray before the baby's conception. This reasoning applies to dental X rays, too. Before pregnancy occurs, a woman ought to visit her dentist and have all necessary dental work completed. That way, when she is pregnant, she won't have to worry about the effects of dental X rays, anesthetics, or laughing gas on her unborn baby. (Having teeth cleaned during pregnancy should be harmless.)

A mother who wants to have her baby at home may have a hard time finding a doctor who will provide medical supervision during her pregnancy. In fact, the woman who broadcasts her intentions may soon discover that no doctor in her community will give her an appointment.

The unanimous refusal of local doctors to provide prenatal care to such women has caused the opening of several
birth centers. These groups have sprung up not to promote
home delivery, but because the people who wanted and
planned home births found themselves involuntarily cut off
from medical care. When local physicians have refused to
provide prenatal care, people who badly need it have had to
start birth groups to get their own.

If couples announce their desire to have their babies at
home, they should face an unpleasant fact. In most areas of
the United States, it will be nearly impossible for them to get
prenatal care. If no alternate source of health care is available,
such as a birth center or women's health group, and the
couple must seek conventional prenatal care, they should
probably keep quiet about their plans to have home childbirth.

A good doctor can sometimes be selected by calling the
local medical society. Ask to be referred to a doctor who
practices natural or family-centered childbirth.

Another way to find a doctor is to call or visit hospitals
which have maternity wards. Often, a hospital receptionist has
some idea of which birth methods are used there. If not, she
may let you talk to someone on the maternity ward. A nurse
who works in the labor and delivery rooms is in an excellent
position to observe whether a doctor encourages family-
centered childbirth or practices the "knock-'em-out,
drag-'em-out" method. Make sure she understands that you
are not asking her for a recommendation, but merely seeking
information.

In most cities, this will involve very few telephone calls.
Due to our falling birthrate, even fairly large cities may have
only three or four hospitals whose maternity wards are still
open.

In very large cities, such as New York or Philadelphia,
there may be a maternity center. This would be an excellent
source of prenatal care. Some women may be eligible for free

prenatal care from outpatient clinics of large hospitals. These offer completely adequate medical supervision, plus care that may prove to be relatively "hassle-free."

"Obstetricians usually do have strong personal and professional needs to control the circumstances of their patients," remarks Dr. John B. Franklin, chief of staff at Philadelphia's Booth Maternity Center.

As a result, some women who could afford the most costly private care prefer to come to such metropolitan maternity centers. A socially prominent countess who had her second baby at Booth said she did so because of doctor disenchantment. During her first pregnancy, she found her private obstetrician frustrating to deal with; while never openly refusing her requests for natural childbirth, he never really committed himself, either.

"My doctor had a sort of professional patter; I felt as if I were talking to a machine," said the countess. Dr. Franklin, on the other hand, "talked to me like a person."[5]

It might be a good idea for a woman to bear this in mind if she must look for a doctor in private practice. If the mother-to-be calls a doctor and asks him if he is interested in natural childbirth, or family-centered childbirth, his response should really be enthusiastic. If the obstetrician's enthusiasm is carefully qualified, the mother should be on the alert for further clues. Here are a few of the things doctors may say about natural childbirth.

> "Of course, it's not for everyone. Not all women are suitable for it."
>
> "The *doctor* has to be the one to decide whether a woman is a good candidate for natural childbirth."
>
> "I don't like patients who insist on natural childbirth because they tie my hands. I must have complete freedom to exercise my professional judgment."
>
> "A woman's relationship with her obstetrician can be even more important than her relationship with her husband. She has to trust him completely."

Attitudes like these caused the author of *Free and Female* to conclude that "many, if not most, American gynecologists are reluctant to go along with natural childbirth under any circumstances."[6]

If there are so few doctors who will even go along with natural childbirth, why should a woman who wants a home delivery bother looking for one? Simply because it's worth it. The doctor who believes in drug-free delivery will be the doctor who is less likely to dictate to his patients on other aspects of prenatal care, such as gaining weight. Also, an obstetrician who tries to avoid using drugs during labor will probably be less likely to prescribe amphetamines, diuretics, and tranquilizers for the various problems of pregnancy. Furthermore, a physician who is open-minded on childbirth *methods* is more likely to be open-minded on childbirth *locations*. Once a pregnant woman has established a good relationship with such a doctor, she may feel free to discuss her feelings about childbirth at home. Most doctors who practice only conventional childbirth, however, will probably not be too receptive to their patients' individual ideas about delivery styles.

Once a woman finds a source of prenatal care, she will usually receive instructions on things like diet and exercise. When it comes to maternal weight gain, even the experts disagree. The expectant mother is usually advised to gain less than eighteen pounds. Yet a few American doctors are beginning to believe that women could gain up to twice that much. Moreover, such large weight gains have been proved to benefit their babies, not harm them.

Mothers who gained less than fifteen pounds during pregnancy were three times as likely to have brain-damaged children and three times as likely to have low-birthweight infants as women who gained thirty-six or more pounds during pregnancy. This was discovered by the Collaborative Study of Cerebral Palsy after an analysis of more than 55,000 births at 14 leading medical centers.[7]

Babies who weigh less than five and one-half pounds at birth are more likely to have lower I.Q.s, malformations, infections, anemia and diarrhea. Babies who weigh over seven and one-half pounds at birth, however, tend to be healthier, smarter and happier; they also develop better during their first year of life. According to a study of thousands of newborns' birth weights sponsored by the National Institute of Health, the larger, superior babies were directly connected to improved maternal diets and weight gains of twenty-five pounds or more. (Although the mothers who ate well had babies who averaged eight and one-half pounds, their deliveries were quite easy. The undernourished mothers' babies averaged less than six pounds, but their births were usually longer and more difficult.)

In 1970, a young California woman was told by her doctor to avoid salt, milk and eggs during her pregnancy. In order to help her keep her weight gain under fifteen pounds, the doctor prescribed diuretic pills for three months. The baby weighed less than five pounds at birth and was "obviously mentally retarded."

Later, this mother was cared for by Dr. Thomas Brewer, whom some people describe as "the Ralph Nader of obstetrics." Under Dr. Brewer's prenatal course, she ate well, gained fifty pounds, and gave birth to a normal baby who weighed almost ten pounds and who was a full six inches longer than her first baby. Comments Dr. Brewer:

> We will continue to have iatrogenic [doctor-caused] malnutrition in human prenatal care until the ACOG recognizes the role of malnutrition in damaging mother and fetus—until we set up some national nutrition standards for human pregnancy nutrition . . .[8]

What types of food does Dr. Brewer tell his patients to eat? In one of his booklets for pregnant mothers, he recommends a daily diet which includes the following foods:

1. 1 quart of milk
2. 2 eggs
3. 1 or 2 additional servings of protein
4. 1 or 2 servings of fresh green leafy vegetables
5. 2 or 3 slices of whole wheat bread
6. 1 orange or cup of orange juice
7. 1 pat of vitamin A-enriched margarine

Let's Have Healthy Children recommends a similar prenatal diet, as does a pamphlet published by the National Dairy Council and approved by the Council on Foods and Nutrition of the A.M.A. This pamphlet indicates, however, that a pregnant woman who is not suffering from a previous nutritional deficiency can get by with one and one-half pints of milk and one egg a day, in addition to the rest of the items on Dr. Brewer's list. Also, besides the citrus fruit or juice, another fresh fruit should be eaten daily. In addition to green vegetables, yellow or orange-colored vegetables like carrots should be eaten five times a week. Whole-grain cereals, such as oatmeal or Wheatena, should be eaten four times a week, and potatoes should also be included.

Recent research suggests that potatoes should be handled with care by pregnant women. In 1972, a London geneticist discovered that women who eat blighted potatoes during the early months of pregnancy have a higher chance of having babies with spina bifida and anencephaly. These are birth defects which prevent complete formation or closing of the spine and the top of the head. In Ireland, where expectant mothers eat many potatoes, the incidence of these birth defects is highest. In southern Japan, where expectant mothers eat very few potatoes, the birth defects only occur in 8 babies out of 10,000. Furthermore, blight is more apt to occur in rainy climates. In both Canada and the United States, the incidence of spina bifida and anencephaly is higher in the east, which has a wetter climate and therefore produces more blighted potatoes.

Pregnant women could cut down on the possibility of

fetal damage by eating only Idaho potatoes. Also, when cooking them, they should discard completely any potato with a brown or black-colored bruise, and avoid breathing the vapors that come from boiling potatoes. Since even one contaminated potato can infect an entire lot, as in mashed potatoes, a pregnant woman can eat them more safely if she boils her own potatoes separately. Also, she should avoid eating any potatoes not prepared by herself.[9]

Does a pregnant woman need extra vitamins? Once again, there is no lack of disagreement among the experts. Many doctors say that a good diet will supply all the nutrients needed by the unborn baby. Nutritional researchers are apt to counter that many of our foods are so highly processed that little real food value remains. So prenatal vitamins may be necessary to prevent deficiencies.

Along with prenatal vitamins, iron pills are usually prescribed for pregnant women. Several nutritionists have pointed out that one of the most commonly prescribed iron tablets, ferrous sulfate, destroys vitamin E in the body. Iron salts are also tolerated only with difficulty by many mothers. Ferrous lactate or ferrous gluconate pills may be acceptable substitutes. Women who have a hard time tolerating these forms of iron might ask their doctors to prescribe a sustained-release form of iron, such as Ferro-Sequels capsules. (They are more expensive, though.)

Many doctors agree that iron from food can be used more easily by the body than iron from supplements. Liver, brewers' yeast, meat, greens, legumes, molasses, dried fruits, and whole grains are beneficial foods that are rich in iron. If a pregnant woman eats them frequently, she builds up the red blood cells which supply oxygen to her unborn baby.

In 1974, Dr. Benjamin Feingold, a noted allergist, testified before a California state committee on the problems of hyperactivity in school children about the role of artificial foods. Noting that hyperactivity was causing learning difficulties and behavior problems in up to ten million American children, Dr. Feingold put the blame on artificial additives. Frequently, when artificially colored or flavored foods have been removed from the diets of hyperactive children, they have dramatically improved within a few days.

Noting that his findings represent what is probably "just the tip of the iceberg," Dr. Feingold called for more research on the effects of synthetic foods on the newborn and unborn baby.[10]

A health research group directed by Ralph Nader exposed more of this particular iceberg. The group recently declared that a widely used food dye, Red 2, is alarmingly and unnecessarily dangerous. In fact, they had asked the F.D.A. to ban its use in 1971. Unfortunately, it's difficult to avoid Red 2, since it's used to color lipstick, pill coatings, Jell-O, ice cream and soft drinks. But even a relatively small amount can be hazardous. According to the Nader group, "if a 110-pound pregnant woman drinks more than a third of a can of strawberry soda pop a day, she risks either cancer or damaging her baby."[11]

Almost every week, researchers discover more teratogens, or agents that can cause harm to an unborn baby. To an expectant mother, it may almost seem as if nothing is safe to eat anymore. In an age when even chemicals found in drinking water are suspect, many women wonder if it's really possible to eat the right things anyway. Nutritional information can be conflicting and confusing; a young mother can easily begin to doubt the value of changing her eating habits. But it *is* worth it. The March of Dimes' *Facts: 1975* confirms that poorly nourished mothers have babies who weigh less, have fewer brain cells, and later learn slowly, even if their diets are improved after birth.

Maximum food value can be obtained if the pregnant woman looks for basic unprocessed foods that have undergone as little refinement as possible. She should eat fresh meats, avoiding hot dogs, luncheon meats, and other factory-cured meat products which contain greater amounts of nitrates. Fresh fruits and vegetables should be chosen. If they are unavailable or too expensive, frozen ones are preferable to canned. (Canned fruits and vegetables lose much of their nutritional value because of the high temperatures used to process them.) Mothers-to-be might experiment with baking whole-grain breads and preparing whole-grain cereals instead of using dry cereals and commercially baked products. Honey can be substituted for white sugar. Cholesterol can be reduced and nutrition boosted by using safflower or corn oil in place of hydrogenated shortening or animal fats. Butter could be replaced by a margarine that lists liquid corn or safflower oil as its first ingredient.

For more detailed information on the reasons behind these recommendations, read *Let's Have Healthy Children,* or *Let's Eat Right to Keep Fit,* both by Adelle Davis. These books also contain a wealth of information on the role of vitamin supplements. Folic acid, for example, can help to prevent birth defects. According to Adelle Davis, women whose urine shows that they lack folic have twice as many deformed babies as women who do not have the folic acid deficiency. When a group of mothers of deformed children were given 5 mg. of folic acid daily during subsequent pregnancies, they all had healthy, normal babies.[12]

Since these amounts of folic acid can be obtained in this country only by prescription, Adelle Davis advises women to ask their doctors to prescribe 1 mg. of folic acid daily during their pregnancies. (Much smaller dosages of folic acid can be found in some health food stores.)

Many physicians tend to scoff at Adelle Davis's recommendations, but new findings often tend to lend them added weight. In 1974, nutritionists at M.I.T. identified folic acid as a nutrient called a lipotrope which helps the unborn baby ward off cancer when he is grown up.

"Combating cancer appears to be in part a function of the thymic-dependent immune system, which is impaired by a lack of the lipotrope nutrient," announced Dr. Paul M. Newberne, professor of nutritional pathology. As a result, his research team recommended that pregnant women who do not have enough of the lipotrope nutrients should have them added to their diets, "or millions of children may later have a harder time warding off infections and diseases."[13]

How many mothers actually suffer from folic acid deficiencies? According to some studies, two out of every three pregnant women in the United States have below-normal levels of this B vitamin.

What about drinking? Most nutritionists recommend that expectant mothers drink three glasses of milk daily, plus water and juice. Coffee and cola drinks contain caffeine, which is believed to dissolve vitamin B, which is then excreted, so they should be eliminated or kept to a bare minimum. Many women switch to iced tea or decaffinated coffee during pregnancy, out of consideration for their babies. Fruit drinks, ices, or popsicles made with artificial coloring and flavoring should be strictly avoided.

Nobody has discovered the unborn child's exact tolerance of liquor, but recent investigations have raised some disturbing questions about it. In Seattle, Washington, researchers studied eight babies born to alcoholic women of different ages and backgrounds. In spite of good food and care *after* they were born, all of the infants suffered permanent adverse effects from their mothers' drinking while they were in the womb. Unusually low I.Q.s, small eye openings, weights little more than one-third of normal, and heights little more than half of normal were shown by all the children. Most of them also had smaller heads and upper jaws than normal; many had heart defects, and some were even born with dislocated hips.[14] Obviously, heavy drinking during pregnancy can inflict severe, undeserved punishment on the unborn child.

Smoking, too, is believed to be harmful to the baby. A 1973 report by the Public Health Service estimated that 4,600 American infants were stillborn each year because their mothers were heavy smokers. (This number is far greater than any of the well-publicized diseases which can endanger the life of the unborn baby.)

The Public Health Service also noted that besides still-births, heavy smoking causes many infants to die just after they are born. If the mother's smoking does not endanger her baby to this extent, he may be smaller and weigh less than he should at birth.[15]

"The number of cigarettes that can be safely smoked by a pregnant woman is *zero*," concludes Dr. Deliveria-Papadopoulas, a clinical researcher at the University of Pennsylvania. When she took blood samples from newborn infants at birth, she found that the babies born to mothers who smoked two packs of cigarettes a day had almost four times the carbon monoxide in their blood as the babies of nonsmokers.[16] Besides, newborn infants whose mothers are heavy smokers often suffer excruciating withdrawal symptoms during their first days of life.

Anything that cuts down the oxygen reaching the fetus harms it. Besides smoking, air pollution, heavy traffic, smoke-filled rooms and cars can all affect the unborn baby adversely. Even holding the breath decreases the fetal oxygen supply. Mothers-to-be who enjoy swimming should continue to do so, but forgo the underwater swims and diving stunts that require prolonged breath holding.

The baby will also get more oxygen if his mother gets some kind of exercise every day. Moderate exercise actually helps to *feed* the baby, too, as it increases the flow of nutrients in the mother's blood through the placenta.

Exercise benefits the mother, as well. It improves her general health, builds up her resistance, prepares her for labor, and tones her perineal muscles so she will be less likely to tear them during delivery.

What is the best exercise during pregnancy? Whatever type of exercise that the woman is used to. Pregnancy is not a good time to take up any new strenuous sport, however, such as tennis or gymnastics. Some obstetricians advise their patients to avoid horseback riding, bowling, skiing, and skating.

Such prohibitions make sense, especially during the latter half of pregnancy. As the baby grows, the mother's center of gravity shifts. When this affects her sense of balance, she is much more likely to fall and injure the unborn child, or stimulate labor prematurely.

Walking, bike riding, swimming, and jogging are safe forms of exercise that can be of benefit, as long as they are not indulged in to the point of exhaustion. Wearing the right clothes can make exercising more enjoyable, too. Especially during the last three months of pregnancy, supporting the breasts and abdomen will help to prevent fatigue. A maternity girdle is not very helpful because the pouch in the front doesn't suppo the baby. A regular girdle does a much better job; buy one that is one size too large and put it on early in the morning. The help it provides in carrying an extra twenty pounds can make all the difference in the world.

Many women with beautiful legs are understandably upset when they develop ugly varicose veins during pregnancy. Since there is no cure except surgery, preventing them would seem well worth the effort. Varicosities can be either reduced or prevented by wearing support stockings throughout pregnancy and by cutting off the leg cuffs on panty-style girdles. (Supp-hose makes pretty, long-lasting pantyhose.) Whatever cuts down blood circulation in the legs should be avoided. On an automobile trip, for example, stop at least every two hours and walk around. If you really have to sit for a long time, elevate your feet if possible. If you can't, change position as frequently as you are able.

Hemorrhoids are varicose veins of the rectum or anus. They frequently occur during pregnancy because the extra weight of the baby impedes the circulation. When a woman stands during the latter part of pregnancy, her perineal and rectal muscles must support much of the weight of the baby; they may become swollen and predisposed to hemorrhoids. Constipation and straining may push the enlarged vein out. The hemorrhoid is then said to be thrombosed; typically, it bleeds, stings, and makes life miserable for its owner!

Birth Book recommends several herbal remedies for the relief of pain from hemorrhoids. A thrombosed hemorrhoid, however, needs medical attention. Ask the doctor to prescribe Anusol or another brand of hemorrhoidal suppositories. Eating 25 milligrams of vitamin B_6 at each meal also ought to help make the problem disappear quickly, according to *Let's Have Healthy Children.*

Once the hemorrhoids are reduced, increased fluids, fresh fruits and vegetables, molasses, wheat germ, and other foods rich in vitamin B will help to prevent them from swelling up again. Only the birth of the baby, however, will completely eliminate the proclivity of expectant mothers to hemorrhoids. In the meantime, frequent rest breaks with the feet elevated should alleviate the strain on the susceptible tissues.

In our current zeal for aerobic exercises, it seems as if calisthenics have been all but forgotten. But during pregnancy they can be more valuable than at almost any other time. They help the mother prepare both body and mind for the approaching birth. Deep knee bends and squatting exercises are invaluable for American women; since we don't usually squat to move our bowels, it's hard for us to feel comfortable in this position. Yet squatting is the way most women in the world have their babies, and physiologically it may be the best position, since it shortens and widens the pelvic outlet.

Perineal tightening exercises and the pelvic rock can improve the muscle tone of the vaginal opening. Furthermore, the woman who is faithful to these exercises learns to gain conscious control over these muscles. This usually helps to prevent tearing of the perineum, since she can "hold in" if the baby's head is born too quickly. (This knack can provide some pleasant surprises for the woman's sexual partner, too.)

Calisthenic exercises don't have to become a dull routine. Rhythmical music makes them much more fun. Records or tapes by the Beatles, Herbie Mann, or Chet Atkins offer good sounds to exercise to. It also helps to get properly "suited up." A colorful leotard or bodysuit makes exercising more comfortable and more pleasant. Almost every book on pregnancy and birth contains pictures and exercise directions, from Grantly Dick-Read's *Childbirth Without Fear* in 1944 to Caterine Milinaire's *birth* in 1974.

Women who are able to attend prepared or natural childbirth classes may get plenty of exercise help from them. Furthermore, most Lamaze and Bradley classes teach relaxation and breathing exercises. Many people don't see why an expectant mother needs to learn how to relax. But anyone who has ever spent a sleepless night will agree that fear, pain, or tension can make it impossible to relax. A woman in labor usually suffers from all three of these, but she can learn ways to relax in spite of them.

"A woman learns how to give birth in the same way that she learns how to swim or write or read," said Dr. Fernand Lamaze, the French obstetrician who popularized the psychoprophylactic method of childbirth. In 1951, he visited Russian hospitals and learned that Pavlov's conditioning principles could be used by women in labor; their use was so widespread in the U.S.S.R. that more than 90 percent of Russian mothers needed no pain relievers at all. According to Dr. Lamaze, if a mother knows how to inhibit the pain signals her body sends to her brain, she will give birth successfully, without pain. When she is able to relax and to breathe properly, she can prevent her brain from experiencing the uterine contractions as painful.

"If a woman fails to adapt, above all, if the respiratory response fails to appear quickly enough to offer compensation, then there follows a quickening of the pulse, breathlessness, tiredness and perhaps even collapse," warned Dr. Lamaze. But training can help the woman to handle the contractions efficiently, as the success of the psychoprophylactic method proves. The Lamaze method of childbirth is used in Russia, in France, and in some parts of China. Wherever it's used in China, the mothers need few or no drugs to relieve pain, and the maternity wards are calm and peaceful. In the Chinese hospitals which still use the conventional methods of childbirth, however, the traditional screams and pandemonium prevail.

If a mother-to-be can't join a prenatal class, she can get most of the benefits by reading. Intelligent research can also help couples make an informed decision about methods of childbirth and about where to have their babies. Probably the best, most balanced book is *Commonsense Childbirth,* by maternity educator Lester D. Hazell. One reason Mrs. Hazell's book has been so popular is that, as an anthropologist, she avoids the extremes of hysteria and pomposity which are apt to creep into even the better books by doctors.

A book which is valuable for anyone considering childbirth at home is lay midwife Raven Lang's *Birth Book.* It contains picture stories of twelve home births, a history of the Santa Cruz home birth movement, instructions, and philosophy. In a unique way of presenting a timeworn subject, each birth story is written by the mother, then told by the father, and finally annotated by the birth attendant. While some of the illustrations may seem almost unbearably graphic, they testify as to the beauty and alertness of the born-at-home babies. And they show very concretely how much the father's help means during labor and delivery.

Several other positive books on birth are listed below in alphabetical order.

Bean, Constance A. *Methods of Childbirth.* New York: Doubleday, 1972.
This is an excellent book to read first. It compares delivery methods and styles from a sociological point of view. The author's scientific objectivity doesn't prevent her from reaching a solid conclusion on the merits of natural childbirth.

Bradley, Robert A. *Husband-Coached Childbirth.* New York: Harper & Row, 1965 and 1974.
Dr. Bradley has been a pioneer in popularizing real

natural childbirth in America; his book includes insights, evaluations, and conclusions derived from thousands of drug-free deliveries.

Chabon, Irwin. *Awake and Aware.* New York: Delacorte, 1966.
This is Dr. Chabon, a New York obstetrician, explains the Lamaze method of psychoprophylactic birth. His well-reasoned arguments rest on a fascinating history of childbirth precedents and practices.

Kitzinger, Sheila. *The Experience of Childbirth.* New York: Taplinger, 1962.
This is the oldest book on the list, but the author's warmhearted common sense makes it still worth reading. Mrs. Kitzinger is a famous British childbirth educator and anthropologist. Her book contains a wealth of well-organized material on home birth.

Liley, H.M.I. and Beth Day. *Modern Motherhood.* New York: Random House, 1969.
Obstetrician Liley explains why mothers should not push during labor. This book presents one of the best explanations of the physiology of labor and delivery.

Tanzer, Deborah and Jean L. Block, *Why Natural Childbirth?* New York: Doubleday, 1972.
A psychologist examines, among other things, the impact of family-centered birth on the personality, contrasting it with the psychological damage often suffered after conventional birth.

White, Gregory J. *Emergency Childbirth.* Franklin Park, Ill. Police Training Foundation, 1968.
This manual tells laymen how to cope with a sudden, normal birth. It teaches natural birth assistance in easy-to-understand language.

NOTES

1. Elliott H. McCleary, *New Miracles of Childbirth* (New York: David McKay, 1974), p. 19.
2. Lloyd Shearer, "Drugs and Pregnancy," *Parade*, January 12, 1975, p. 15.
3. Caterine Milinaire, *birth* (New York: Harmony Books, 1974), p. 51.
4. Virginia Apgar, M.D., and Joan Beck, *Is My Baby All Right?* (New York: Trident Press, 1972), p. 103.
5. Judy Klemesrud, "Why Women Are Losing Faith in Their Doctors," *McCalls*, June 1973, p. 105.
6. Barbara Seaman, *Free and Female* (New York: Coward, McCann & Geoghegan, Inc., 1972), p. 141.
7. Elliott H. McCleary, op. cit., p. 58.
8. Ibid., p. 56.
9. Ibid., p. 33.
10. Arlene Hetherington, "Sickening Diet," *The Sacramento Bee*, December 16, 1974, p. B3.
11. "Nader Warns Food Dye Is Dangerous," *The Sacramento Bee*, November 1, 1974, p. A5.
12. Adelle Davis, *Let's Have Healthy Children* (New York: Harcourt Brace Jovanovich, 1972), p. 32.
13. "Mother's Diet Sets Disease Defenses," *The Sacramento Bee*, September 7, 1974, p. A5.
14. Ellen Crane, "What's New in Medicine" (Alcoholism and Birth Defects) *Lady's Circle*, July 1974, p. 45.
15. "Medicine Today," *Ladies Home Journal*, September 1973, p. 26.
16. Elliott H. McCleary, op. cit., p. 60.

OTHER SOURCES

Sheldon H. Cherry, M.D., *Understanding Pregnancy and Childbirth* (Indianapolis: Bobbs-Merrill, 1973.)

Boston Women's Health Book Collective, Inc., *Our Bodies, Ourselves* (New York: Simon & Schuster, 1973.)

Thomas Brewer, M.D., *If You Are Pregnant and Want Your Child . . .* (Berkeley, California: Student Research Facility.)

National Foundation/March of Dimes, *Facts: 1975*.

Grantly Dick-Read, *Childbirth Without Fear* (New York: Harper & Row, 1944.)

Fernand Lamaze, M.D., *Painless Childbirth: The Psychoprophylactic Method* (New York: Henry Regnery Company, 1970.)

Raven Lang, *Birth Book* (Ben Lomond, California: Genesis Press, 1972.)

8

WHAT TO DO ON BABY'S "BIRTH DAY"

Commonsense Childbirth and other books say that advance planning makes the difference between a successful home delivery and one that just happens; the couple expecting a baby should make plans for its birth several weeks in advance. Hopefully, the husband and wife have already found out what options are available to them in their local community; ideally, they have read enough material on birth so they can evaluate these options. If they have decided to have their baby at home, they should make the necessary preparations about a month before the baby is due. (If the birth occurs before this, the premature baby will probably need specialized care, and plans for home delivery should be abandoned.)

"If you go into labor six weeks or more before due date," advises Dr. John Grausz of Milwaukee County Hospital, "don't bother with an inadequate facility. For the sake of the baby and often the mother, forget the community hospital. ... . Call the emergency squad or police and get yourself rushed to the nearest perinatal center, if it's reachable."[1]

Parents-to-be should also head for a hospital or perina-

149

tal center promptly if bright red blood comes from the mother's vagina during the last three months of pregnancy. This may mean that the placenta has begun to detach prematurely. It happens in only a very small number of pregnancies, perhaps one in two hundred, but when it does, expert medical attention may be needed to prevent the mother from hemorrhaging.[2] Also, if possible, the baby should be delivered in a hospital which has all the special equipment to handle premature and high-risk infants. Most perinatal centers are located in metropolitan hospitals which are affiliated with medical schools. Others are part of large county hospitals, such as Los Angeles County-USC Medical Center in California and Milwaukee County Hospital in Wisconsin.

But if everything goes smoothly during pregnancy, the couple who wants a home birth will probably want to start getting ready. As they do so, however, they should make sure the wife continues her prenatal visits to the doctor or clinic. It's important to have medical monitoring right through pregnancy. Besides, often the doctor or midwife can tell when the baby's head drops low in the uterus. This used to be called "lightening"; today the baby is said to be "engaged." Whatever the doctor calls it, the effect on the mother is that the baby's lower position gives her more room to breathe. Also, symptoms of heartburn may disappear, as the baby's weight no longer crowds the mother's stomach. The woman who is told that her baby is engaged can breathe a sigh of relief. He is now in the right position to be born.

(If the full-term baby has *not* dropped into this head-down position, the birth probably shouldn't take place at home. Complications are more frequent in breech births, when the baby is not born head first. To protect their baby's safety, parents who suspect a breech birth ought to forego the luxury of a home delivery.)

Couples who plan to go ahead with home delivery, however, might do well to take a few of their neighbors and close friends into their confidence. Offers of help should not be declined! If a friend or relative would be willing to come over at the beginning of labor, she could handle the ordinary household tasks so the husband can stay with his wife. It's a good idea to stock up on nourishing food that's easy to prepare. Some women like to bake and freeze a cake for the coming "birth day" celebration.

The couple should make sure that everyone involved knows the exact roles they are going to play. The mother in labor should not find herself in the position of having to act as hostess to a house full of people. If this seems like a potential problem, the couple can explain, *in advance,* that they are having their baby at home because they value their privacy and consider birth as an intimate occasion. To many people, having a baby is as private an act as sexual intercourse. Furthermore, the embarrassment or strain caused by the presence of other people can create tension in the mother and make the birth more difficult. Neighbors can show their consideration, however, by helping in their own homes. They could take in the couple's older children, or fix them a casserole to heat after the baby is born.

A few of the recent books on home delivery show the birth taking place in a room full of people. This is fine, if the mother really wants it that way. Her desires ought to be respected since she is the one who is having the baby.

"At the bedsides of birth and death, kindly company is the best of all commodities," says Dr. H.M.I. Liley in *Modern Motherhood.* Whether a woman wants to have only her husband present, or to enjoy the support of several friends, her preferences should be paramount.

Parents may wonder whether their older children, or their friends' children should be invited to attend a home birth. Dr. Henry Harrison Sadler, a California professor of psychiatry, thinks this depends on the child's age. A toddler under eighteen months old should not have to be excluded from childbirth at home. A child over five years old will probably be mature enough to understand what is happening.

Children between one and a half and five, however, may be adversely affected if they are allowed to witness a home delivery.

Dr. Lee Coleman, a child psychiatrist, thinks that harm could more easily be done to a child who is expected to participate or pressured into seeing a home birth. According to Dr. Coleman, the family should feel comfortable about the birth, and should not push the child into sharing the experience. Otherwise, it could prove destructive to him, emotionally.

The presence of children at a birth is accepted in many cultures, but it is not common in ours, except for a very few enclaves in the western United States. It's not surprising, then, that many experts doubt the wisdom of exposing children to an event which might upset them.

"In the limited experience of a child, blood means injury and a strained expression means anger or pain," points out Ms. Thelma Harms of the University of California's Harold E. Jones Child Study Center. "A child might feel frightened seeing his mother in such a vulnerable state. . . . Birth and death are very trying experiences for any age, and they take maturity to handle."[3]

The bed where the baby will be born can be prepared ahead of time. If it's very soft, put a plywood board under the mattress. Then put a plastic sheet or an old shower curtain over the mattress. This will protect it in case the mother's water breaks at night. Cover the plastic sheet with a mattress pad and make up the bed as usual.

To get the birth sheets ready, collect an old sheet, a few old towels, and a crib-sized rubber sheet—the kind that's flannelized. Wash them in hot water, using chlorine bleach. Then tumble-dry them at the highest temperature possible. As soon as the dryer stops, fold the sheets and towels while they are still hot. Put them in an unused plastic bag and keep the bag in a bureau drawer close to the bed.

Toddler-sized disposable diapers can be used instead of

the towels. They will come in handy many times during labor and delivery.

Some books recommend dental floss for tying the umbilical cord, but white shoelaces are much easier to handle. Buy a pair of short ones, or cut a single long one in half. (The baby's cord ought to be tied in two places.) The shoelaces can be sterilized by washing and drying them with the sheets. Put them away separately in an unused plastic sandwich bag.

A large bowl or a baby bathtub should be available for the afterbirth. Any large pot or pan will do, but it should be low enough so that the mother can squat or sit over it comfortably. Blunt-pointed scissors are best for cutting the cord, but ordinary scissors are all right if used with great care. They should be sterilized in boiling water while the mother is in early labor. Later, when you are ready to cut the cord, dip the scissors in rubbing alcohol first.

The most important piece of equipment needed for a home birth is a rubber syringe to aspirate the baby. While most home-born babies breathe spontaneously, a syringe must be available in case yours does not. The type to look for is rubber, with no plastic parts. The business end should be at least one and a half inches long so it can reach deep enough into the baby's throat to remove any mucus which may be lodged there. (In an emergency, a poultry baster could be used for this.)

Don't forget to buy baby clothes and diapers. Wash them, using enough fabric softener so they won't irritate the newborn's skin. Keep a few receiving blankets handy to wrap the baby in as soon as he's born. This is especially important if the house is cool.

Birth Book, Commonsense Childbirth, birth, and others contain itemized lists of things to have on hand for a home delivery. Each one is a little different, so it would probably be best to read them and use them as guides. Items such as cotton swabs (Q-tips) and sanitary napkins will no doubt be convenient, but some couples may think that sterile gloves and antiseptic soap are not strictly necessary. (Of course, nobody who has an infection should consider delivering a baby.)

One book mentions umbilical clamps and explains how to use them. Many people feel that equipment like this should only be used by a doctor or midwife, unless the husband has steady nerves and knows exactly what to do. Umbilical clamps are for an emergency situation only; if the baby's head is born with the cord all wrapped around his neck, there may not be enough of the umbilicus left for his body to be delivered. If the baby is not born with the next contraction, the umbilical clamps can be used so the cord can be cut safely, thus freeing the baby.

The danger is that under the stress of the moment, a father or other inexperienced birth attendant will clamp and cut the cord when there is no real need to do so. Even if the umbilical cord is wrapped around the baby's neck, in most cases it can be slipped over his head and the birth can proceed normally.

These unusual possibilities do not have to concern the couple who is fortunate enough to have found a capable midwife, or other birth attendant. Not only will he or she have the expertise to deal with the unexpected, but the attendant will bring much of the needed equipment. Sometimes, the parents prepare the sheets, towels and bowls, while the mid-wife brings her own scissors, aspirator, and any other surgical supplies.

Many people are afraid that sexual activity near the end of pregnancy will harm the baby or start labor prematurely. It won't. In fact, several authorities say that abstaining from intercourse six weeks before the due date may be harmful to the mother because it makes her depressed and nervous. The mild vaginal contractions which a woman experiences during orgasm help to tone the perineal muscles; a normal sex life helps the mother approach childbirth in a mor relaxed frame of mind. In fact, some societies practice intercourse during the very early stages of labor; they believe it helps the woman relax and promotes an easy delivery.[4]

Normal sexual relations do not bother the baby. In one study of 500 women, those who continued to have intercourse until a few days before birth had no more complications than those who abstained for weeks before birth.[5] Until labor begins, the uterus is sealed by a thick plug of mucus which prevents infections from entering. While the lower part of this cervical plug contains numerous bacteria, the upper part is virtually sterile.[6] Of course, the mother should not have sexual relations after this mucus has come out, or if her waters have broken. Nor should she attempt intercourse if it feels painful.

The loosening and passing out of the cervical plug usually signals the beginning of labor. It's sometimes called the bloody show, since the mucus is tinged with blood. If the mother experiences contractions when she passes the bloody show, it's a good sign that labor has begun in earnest. Some women do not feel real contractions during the very early phase of labor, but they may notice a low backache or a sensation of tightness around the crotch or a feeling of stretching around the abdomen.

If a woman is expecting her first baby and mild labor begins at night, it may be just as well if she tries to get as much sleep as possible during the early stages. If the contractions are disturbing, a heating pad can often help. Aspirin should not be taken though. It can cause bleeding problems in the newborn baby.[7]

If the mother is alone, she should get somebody to be with her, preferably someone who will stay until at least a few hours after the birth. Then she should eat a light but nourishing meal. Digestion stops when the woman is in hard labor, so the meal ought to be taken early. Eating will give the mother strength and make her contractions seem much less painful. A good snack for the beginning of labor might include toast and cheese, fruit, and a glass of milk. Of course, the mother should not force herself to eat, but she should try to take something solid to build up her strength. If she doesn't feel up to tackling the more nutritious foods, Jell-O or cookies would be better than nothing.

Adelle Davis advises taking extra vitamin E and C at the onset of labor, and sipping fortified Pep-up every three hours thereafter. There is much evidence to suggest that Vitamin E, folic acid, Vitamin C, pantothenic acid, and zinc can help to shorten labor and make the birth safer for both mother and baby. *Let's Have Healthy Children* contains complete information and instructions on nutrition during pregnancy, labor and delivery.

After fortifying herself with a snack, the mother should try to empty her bowels to make room for the baby's descent. Many women experience a "normal" diarrhea before labor starts, so they don't have to do anything to help nature along. If a woman's bowels have not moved recently, however, she could take two tablespoonfuls of castor oil and drink a small glass of orange juice. This will usually produce results in well under a half an hour. A woman who can't tolerate castor oil can use a glycerine suppository instead. Buy them in a drugstore and follow the directions on the package.

After this, the mother may feel more comfortable if she takes a warm bath. A bath will help her to relax, it helps to increase the circulation of the blood to her stomach, and it often helps to keep the contractions regular. The mother should wash her entire bottom well, using an antibacterial soap. Someone should stay with her in the bathroom all the time, helping her get into and out of the tub.

A shower can be substituted for the bath. It will be just as hygienic, but a bath will do more to actively promote the birth.

When the mother is clean, she should put on a soft, comfortable nightgown or shift and lie down. The bed should be adjusted until she is perfectly comfortable, with the covers loose. Pillows, heating pad, talcum powder, socks and blankets can all be used to make the woman in labor feel at ease. Ideally, labor should take place in a quiet, dimly lit room where she feels completely secure. She may need help to find the best position; moving around can be difficult at this time.

Hopefully, the husband will be actively involved in all these preparations. Once the wife is settled, he can sterilize the infant aspirator and scissors in boiling water. They can be wrapped in a clean towel until later. A small bowl or pan that has been sterilized with boiling water can be filled with alcohol and taken to the bedroom. Then it will be handy to dip the aspirator, scissors and shoelaces in when they are needed.

During labor, the husband can offer his wife sips of water, help her go to the bathroom every hour, rub her back, and tell her how great she's doing. Mostly, he can help by just *being* there to calm her and respond to her needs. If she seems to need more than reassurance to help handle her contractions, the husband can fix her a drink.

Spikenard tea, pukeweed tea, and a multitude of other folk remedies have been recommended for labor through the ages. Alcohol, however, seems to have stood the test of time very well. During active labor, the mother's metabolism works so rapidly that there is little danger of her getting drunk. This speeded-up metabolism also helps to insure that the liquor she ingests won't depress the unborn baby.

If she wants it, the mother can be given a mixed drink with ice, using a sweet carbonated drink to dilute the alcohol. Ginger ale or cola is ideal because it soothes the stomach. Also, the sugar in it gives the mother extra energy during labor. Kentucky straight bourbon whisky mixes well with ginger ale, according to generations of mothers!

If the woman does not like the idea of hard liquor during labor, she might prefer wine. Wine is a pleasant and effective tranquilizer which has promoted relaxation since antiquity. Besides, wine supplies vitamins, minerals, iron and sugar—all of which will be quickly utilized by a mother undergoing the rigors of labor.

Just how bad is the pain of childbirth? *Why Natural Childbirth?* compares labor to the pain caused by third-degree burns or physical torture. There is no doubt that birth can be extremely painful. But fear, fatigue, tension, loneliness, cold, and hunger or thirst all increase the severity of pain. So does an uncomfortable position. The woman whose contractions are uncomfortable can alleviate them by relaxing and getting into a position which eases them. Of course, the normal reaction to pain is to tense the muscles to fight it. But during labor, this only forces the uterus to work harder and causes even more pain. If the mother can relax, breathe deeply, and let go of the muscles in her abdomen and pelvic floor, her uterus will be able to effect the birth more quickly and efficiently.

The discomfort of labor is caused when the uterus contracts, pressing itself against the cervix, and opening it little by little until it thins and separates enough to let the baby's head enter the vagina. This explains why the first labor is almost always the longest. After the cervix has been dilated by the birth of one child, subsequent labors may be experienced as only a few mild cramps.[8]

A woman who has a small, tight cervix should probably be prepared to endure real pain during labor. A usually reliable indicator is her menstrual history. Women who have irregular periods characterized by acute cramps at their onset tend to have significantly more childbirth pain than women who menstruate regularly with little or no disturbance of their daily activities.[9] Studies have shown that natural childbirth techniques can help mothers with good menstrual histories escape serious birth pains completely. A woman with a tight cervix can *reduce* her pain by using these methods, but she probably should not expect them to be a panacea. An understanding, supportive husband who offers a few sips of a highball will help to see her through the most difficult contractions.

Estimates differ widely on how long labor should last. An average labor for a first baby is about fifteen hours, but longer labors are not uncommon.[10] (If a mother labors at home for more than twenty-four hours without the birth being imminent, she should be taken to a hospital.) In *Maternal Emotions,* Dr. Niles Newton points out that normal, first-time mothers who are well-prepared for natural childbirth can deliver their babies in less than nine hours.[11] Subsequent deliveries, of course, require much less time—on occasion, less than an hour.

People often wonder whether the first baby should be born at home. In England, where many babies are born at home, mothers are asked to go to the hospital for their first delivery. Several American doctors and midwives who attend home births, however, think that emergencies are more likely to occur during subsequent births. They say that the muscles of a young woman who has never had a baby are far more elastic. As a result, less bleeding and fewer complications may be expected following the birth of a first baby.

Perhaps the greatest deterrent to home births for first babies is the possibility that the long labor usually associated with them may make the mother feel discouraged. Being prepared for it will help to avoid this. Also, the superior relaxation which home birth promotes can sometimes cause even a first baby to arrive more quickly than expected.

At the end of the first stage of labor, many mothers experience confusion and a temporary loss of equilibrium. They may become angry, impatient, or suddenly sleepy. Sweating, trembling, or even vomiting may occur. This is the hardest part of labor. It's caused by the baby's head trying to enter the birth canal, pressing against the almost-completely-dilated cervix. Contractions may lose their regular rhythm. The woman may get a sudden low backache as the baby's head finally slips down and puts pressure against her tailbone.

The mother needs soothing assistance more than ever during transition. The husband can massage her back deeply to counteract the internal pain. He can offer his wife ice chips or sour balls to suck on, but she should have nothing else to eat or drink until after the baby is born. If the woman has chills, socks or a heating pad may help. Most of all, the husband should continue to encourage her to relax and to breathe deeply. It's not time to push yet.

"Continued forceful pushing against an incompletely dilated cervix can make it puffy and swollen so that the opening, instead of getting wider for the baby's head to come through, is actually made smaller, and labour is held up," according to Kitzinger's *The Experience of Childbirth*. Besides, pushing before the right time will make the contractions feel much more painful.

If the mother has a chance, the husband should encourage her to empty her bladder, so the baby will have as much room as possible. Should the contractions be too close together, instead of going to the bathroom, she can use a bedpan, a kitchen pot, or even a towel. It's important to keep the bladder empty; try to take care of this every hour or two throughout labor.

The contractions which expel the baby cause the mother much less internal pain than the first-stage contractions which dilate the cervix. After the beginning of the second stage, the birth can take place any time from about ten minutes until two hours. The husband or birth attendant might try to help the wife get into a more upright position. It seems to expedite delivery if the mother can sit or squat. The husband can support her or she can brace herself against pillows.

During the second stage of labor, the uterine contractions work to force the baby down the birth canal and out into the world. The mother can help by pushing with them. She should only push if it feels right. Often, she will be able to tell because pushing will make her feel better. If the woman's expulsive efforts make the contractions feel worse, she should *not* push. Instead, she should continue to relax, leaving the uterus to its own devices.

From the time that the mucus plug comes out, only a

slight amount of blood should be seen during labor. A steady flow of blood before the baby's birth is a sign of some complication; the mother should be taken to a hospital right away. In order to minimize the blood loss, the laboring woman ought to assume the knee-chest position during the trip.

Another indication of danger is a change in the color of the amniotic waters during labor. If they don't look clear, the baby may be in distress. If the mother can't get the baby born soon, she should go to the hospital. (Complications like these are extremely rare at a home birth, but parents ought to be aware of them—especially if their baby is born with no birth attendant present.)

Never try to break the bag of waters during labor. Although this is a routine practice in most hospitals, it increases the possibility of infection and makes the infant's head more vulnerable to disalignment of the parietal bones. Besides cushioning the baby's skull during labor, the amniotic fluid helps to prevent the umbilical cord from becoming compressed. This insures a steadier flow of oxygen to the infant as he descends through the birth canal.[12]

When the husband or birth attendant sees the top of the baby's head during contractions, he should scrub his hands with antibacterial soap and hot water and sterilize the rubber syringe. He can then massage his wife's perineum between contractions. This will help to stimulate circulation in the perineal area and avoid tearing the mother.* Perineal massage can be done with an oil rich in vitamin E, such as wheat germ oil, or a vitamin-enriched cream. K-Y jelly or Vaseline would be all right, too.

When the mother feels a burning, stretching sensation, the baby's head is pressing against her perineum and birth is imminent. The mother should stop pushing, lean back, and go completely limp. It's especially important that she let go of the muscles of the pelvic floor, as tensing them at this time can

* In fact, many midwives advise the couple to practice perineal massage throughout the last month of pregnancy.

cause a perineal tear. The father can really help most by telling his wife what's going on as her labor reaches its climax.

Don't do anything else until the baby's head is born. Never pull on the head; it's not necessary to support the baby's head, either. When the head is born, the attendant can suck mucus from his throat, if the baby is not already crying. With the next contraction, the mother can push gently to rotate the baby's body. Usually the rest of the baby will then slide out smoothly. If not, wait until the next contraction pushes out the baby's top shoulder. Then, you can ease the baby upwards so the bottom shoulder is born slowly. The mother should not push, for suddenly delivering both shoulders at once can make her tear.

When the baby is born, hold his head down low, face down, while you suction mucus from his throat, mouth, and nose. Don't worry about the outer areas; put the aspirator back in his throat where thick mucus may be stuck. If the baby is crying clearly, of course you don't have to do such a scrupulous job with the syringe. Keep the baby lower than the mother for a few moments, so that he can get as much oxygen and nutrients as possible from the placenta. Then wrap him loosely in a warm blanket and let the mother hold him. Relax!

There is no hurry about cutting the umbilical cord. Doctors and midwives who attend many home deliveries say it's better to wait until the afterbirth is born before cutting the cord. In the meantime, the mother's abdomen should be massaged until the uterus feels as firm as a grapefruit. She can do this herself. In about ten or fifteen minutes, the mother may feel a contraction and a slight gush of blood. This means that the placenta is starting to detach itself from the uterus. Support the mother while she sits or squats to deliver the placenta.

The delivery of the placenta, or afterbirth, is sometimes called the third stage of labor. It's expelled by uterine contractions just like the baby. The mother can help to deliver it by pushing with the mild contractions. If she doesn't feel any, standing and stretching may help. Allowing the baby to nurse will often stimulate the uterus to contract and expel the placenta, too.

The afterbirth should be laid flat and examined. Any place where it has torn should fit together with another place, like a jigsaw puzzle. If there is a piece of the placenta missing, it may still be in the uterus. This can cause serious bleeding, so the mother should be taken to a hospital for it to be removed. Also, if the afterbirth has not been delivered within two hours after the baby's birth, medical help should be sought.

When the placenta is out, the umbilical cord can be tied and cut. (If the afterbirth takes its time, the cord can be cut before, as long as it has stopped pulsating completely.) First, dip the clean shoelaces, string, or dental floss in alcohol. Tie the first shoelace securely around the cord about an inch from the baby. Then tie the other one an inch outside the first. Make sure the knots are tight; you can wrap the shoelaces around twice to make them more secure. Then dip the scissors in alcohol and cut the cord between the two knots. Be sure not to poke the baby with the points of the scissors.

The husband should stay with the mother and baby constantly for at least an hour after the birth. It's a good idea for the doctor or midwife to remain that long, too. Someone should massage the mother's uterus gently so that it stays contracted and blood clots are expelled.

People often wonder whether they should take the mother to a hospital for stitches, if she tears during the birth. The great majority of perineal tears suffered during home deliveries are superficial and heal by themselves. Women who have exercised conscientiously may not tear at all. Out of the first eighty-seven home births recorded by the Santa Cruz Birth Center, seventy mothers either didn't tear at all or tore only very superficially.

If the tear is more than a half an inch long, however, or if it is deep, it will heal better with a stitch or two. A doctor can come to the house and put them in, or the mother can be taken to the nearest hospital.

If your town has a Visiting Nurses Association that provides maternity care, call them as soon as possible after the birth. When the nurse arrives, she will examine the perineum for tears and help decide whether stitches are advisable. She will also be able to tell whether the mother would benefit from medication to help her uterus contract.

Even if the mother feels fine, she should rest quietly for the first few hours after the birth. Fever, pallor, or excess bleeding are warning signals; if the woman does not look normal, she should be taken to the hospital. Keep the number of an ambulance service handy and don't hesitate to call one immediately if medical help may be needed. The danger of postpartum hemorrhaging cannot be ignored. It's all right for the woman to lose a cup or two of blood during childbirth, but a sudden gush of bright red blood is a danger sign. If this should happen, and there is no time to wait for help to arrive, the mother can be taken to a hospital by car. During the trip, she should lie down with her feet elevated higher than her head.

Although the first hour after birth is more critical for the mother, the baby should be closely watched, too. If you hear mucus rattling in his throat, use the aspirator to gently suction it out. Keep an eye on the tied-off cord; make sure that blood doesn't seep from it. Watch for the baby to urinate and move his bowels. These are signs that all is well with his internal plumbing. (His first few movements will be a black mucoid substance called meconium.)

People who contemplate childbirth at home most frequently wonder what to do if the baby doesn't start breathing by himself. It's reassuring to know that the vast majority of undrugged babies born at home begin crying during or immediately after birth. If the baby does not breathe spontaneously, hold him with his face down and suction the mucus. If the baby's passages are clear but he still doesn't start breathing, lie him on his back and put your hands on his chest. Keep one hand on his heart to make sure it's beating. Massage his chest firmly with the other hand.

As long as there is a heartbeat, keep trying to resuscitate the baby. Don't waste time slapping him or using cool water, though. Begin giving mouth-to-mouth resuscitation, following the directions in *Birth Book* or a Red Cross manual of first aid or lifesaving. Be sure to blow only puffs of air into the infant's lungs; they are small and cannot hold an adult-size breath.

Have someone watch the baby while you perform artificial respiration. If his heart continues and he shows any response, keep on until he starts breathing by himself. Then wrap him up warmly, let the mother hold him, and watch him carefully for any further signs of distress.

Attempts at resuscitation can be abandoned if the baby's heart is not beating or if he shows no response at all. Lack of movement and lack of color are signs that life isn't there. If the pupils of the baby's eyes are dilated so much that you can't see any color, prepare to give up on resuscitating it. Don't go by the clock or worry about how much time has passed. Just observe the infant for clues; if he shows any signs of life, continue breathing for him as long as you have to.

NOTES

1. Elliott H. McCleary, *New Miracles of Childbirth* (New York: David McKay, 1974), p. 156.
2. Caterine Milinaire, *birth* (New York: Harmony Books, 1974), p. 94.
3. Kaye Yost, "At Home Or In The Hospital?" *California Living*, November 3, 1974, p. 9.
4. Sheila Kitzinger, *The Experience of Childbirth* (New York: Taplinger Publishing Company, 1962), p. 72.
5. Boston Children's Medical Center, *Pregnancy, Birth and the Newborn Baby* (Boston: Boston Children's Medical Center, 1971), p. 14.
6. Isidore Bonstein, M.D., *Psychoprophylactic Preparation for Painless Childbirth* (London: Morrison & Gibb, Ltd., 1958), p. 9.
7. Deborah Tanzer, and Jean L. Block, *Why Natural Childbirth?* (Garden City, New York: Doubleday & Company, 1972), p. 50.

8. William J. Sweeney III, M.D., with Barbara Lang Stern, *Woman's Doctor* (New York: William Morrow, 1973), p. 244.
9. Deborah Tanzer, and Jean L. Block, op. cit., p. 157.
10. Raven Lang, *Birth Book* (Ben Lomond, California: Genesis Press, 1972)
11. Niles Newton, M.D., *Maternal Emotions* (New York: Paul E. Hoeber, Inc., 1955), p. 33.
12. Suzanne Arms, "How Hospitals Complicate Childbirth," *Ms.*, May 1975, p. 109.

OTHER SOURCES
(listed as they appear in text)

Lester Dessez Hazell, *Commonsense Childbirth* (New York: G.P. Putnam's Sons, 1969.)

H.M.I. Liley, M.D., and Beth Day, *Modern Motherhood* (New York: Random House, 1969.)

Helen Wessel, *Natural Childbirth and the Family* (New York: Harper & Row, 1973.)

Adelle Davis, *Let's Have Healthy Children* (New York: Harcourt Brace Jovanovich, 1972.)

Robert A. Bradley, M.D., *Husband-Coached Childbirth* (New York: Harper & Row, 1965.)

Nicholson J. Eastman, M.D. and Keith P. Russell, M.D., *Expectant Motherhood* (Boston: Little, Brown & Company, 1970.)

Patricia Cloyd Carter, *Come Gently, Sweet Lucina* (Titusville, Florida: Patricia Cloyd Carter, 1957.)

Frederick W. Goodrich, Jr., M.D., *Preparing for Childbirth* (Englewood Cliffs, N.J.: Prentice-Hall, Inc., 1966.)

Derek Llewellyn-Jones, M.D., *Everywoman and Her Body* (New York: Taplinger Publishing Company, 1971.)

Fernand Lamaze, M.D., *Painless Childbirth: The Psychoprophylactic Method* (New York: Henry Regnery Company, 1970.)

Donna and Rodger Ewy, *Preparation for Childbirth—A Lamaze Guide* (Boulder, Colorado: Pruett Publishing Company, 1970.)

Pierre Vellay, M.D., *Childbirth with Confidence* (New York: Macmillan, 1969.)

Virginia Apgar, M.D. and Joan Beck, *Is My Baby All Right?* (New York: Trident Press, 1972.)

9

AFTER THE BIRTH IS OVER

At last the baby has been born. Nine months of wondering are finally over, as the parents happily contemplate their new little "him" or "her." Euphoria usually dominates the first few hours after a home birth. Father and mother feel free to examine and cuddle their newborn infant as they call their friends and spread the good news. If they have older children, they will be able to share the excitement. To celebrate the new arrival, some families have a "birthday" party, complete with cake and presents for baby's older brothers and sisters.

"Home confinement does not eliminate sibling jealousy, but it can defer its appearance and possibly also lessen its intensity."[1] Childbirth at home seems to make it easier for older brothers and sisters to accept the new baby as a member of the family. Some authorities think this is because the older child has not been deprived of his mother's presence and thus does not blame it on the newborn infant. Others say that home birth removes the mysterious, sometimes frightening implications that a young child may associate with hospitals. If his mother goes to the hospital to have a baby, the toddler may conclude that the birth was a dangerous operation. Anxiety over her condition and resentment about her "desertion" of him add to his feelings of displacement. Often, when mother finally returns from the hospital, the family's attention may be totally focused on the newborn intruder. This situation naturally provides a setting in which the seeds of sibling rivalry take root and grow. Sadly enough, many such children become so overwhelmed by their emotions that the baby must be protected from them. When the baby is born at home, however, these problems usually do not arise.

Caring for the newborn infant is quite simple during the first few days. The white vernix covering his skin may be left on and rubbed in gently. Many people think it has a protective function. Later, the baby may be sponged with warm water or cleaned with warm oil on cotton balls, but he should not be bathed until his cord has dropped off and the scar healed. In the meantime, baby shampoo can be used to wash his hair; this will help to prevent the formation of cradle cap.

It's a good idea to leave the baby at least partly dressed while washing him because taking off his clothes activates his fear of falling.[2] Usually the infant will be less afraid if you leave his shirt on while washing his bottom half. Then you can hold him in a towel, remove his shirt, and wash his face, arms and chest. This method takes no more time, and it greatly diminishes baby's protestations!

It doesn't seem to matter to the baby what kind of clothing he is dressed in, but being wrapped up in a large receiving blanket augments his feelings of security. It's especially important to keep the infant's body temperature up during the first few hours after he is born; he may have trouble breathing if not kept warm enough. The baby's diapers should be pinned low, so they don't irritate the stump of the umbilical cord. Clothing the baby in a long cotton nightgown or romper-suit will help to keep him from breaking the cord off too soon. If there is swelling, bleeding, or discharge from the cord, have a doctor look at it promptly. Otherwise, it should be left alone as much as possible. Dabbing a bit of alcohol on it every day will help it to dry up and fall off. After it drops off, continue swabbing the navel daily with alcohol or antiseptic for about a week until the scar is completely healed.

If no medical attendant has been present during the birth and no visiting nurse has come to check the baby, he should be brought to a pediatrician or clinic for a newborn checkup. The doctor or nurse will examine him and confirm that he's as healthy as he seems. This should not be neglected or postponed; some birth defects, such as cleft palate, need medical attention right away. The pediatric clinic may also provide infant vitamins, fluoride drops, and booklets on newborn baby care.

After the pediatric examination, the baby may be sent to have a PKU test. Phenylketonuria is a rare disease that affects about one person in ten thousand. Commonly, the baby's heel is stabbed with a small stilette and the blood soaked into several circles on a white absorbent card. Not only can this be a traumatic ordeal for both mother and child, but the process is frequently lengthened by the baby's having received a vitamin K shot, which makes his blood coagulate more quickly. The lab technician then has to make repeated stabs on the baby's heel in order to obtain the necessary amount of blood.

State law may force the parents to agree to the PKU test. Some pediatricians, however, think the test results are not completely reliable until the baby is a few weeks old. Also, PKU can sometimes be detected by a simple urine test.[3] It might be advisable to find out beforehand what the clinic's policy is on newborn procedures. At the same time, a couple who is free of gonorrhea can inquire whether their baby's eyes must have silver nitrate or antibiotic treatment. State law may require this, but in some states, the law only applies to babies born in the hospital. The county health agency or state department of health can best explain these regulations.

It's a good idea to allow the baby to nurse at frequent intervals during the first day or two after his birth. *Commonsense Childbirth* explains why·

Babies who have trouble learning to eat are usually the ones who have not been offered their mothers' breasts soon after birth. The nursing instinct is very strong as soon as the baby has his breathing well enough coordinated so that he can suck and swallow and breathe. With most babies that is immediately after birth; with those who have mucus or are drugged, it takes longer; but like many other learning patterns in children, if the sucking desire is thwarted when it first arises, the baby gets discouraged and may have to be taught to suck later.[4]

Mothers who have nursed their babies say it's better not to encourage long periods of sucking for the first few days; this will make the nipples irritated and sore when the milk comes in. There is no need to worry about the baby's health in the meantime. Infants of well-nourished mothers are born with enough stored glycogen to carry them over for several days.[5] Meanwhile, when the baby nurses, he receives colostrum, a yellowish liquid that contains more than twice as much protein as regular breast milk, plus generous amounts of vitamins A and E. After three or four days, this colostrum will gradually be replaced by real breast milk.

"Breast milk is food for infants; cow's milk is food for calves," states a World Health Organization nutritionist. Mother's milk contains exactly the right proportions of nutrients for the human baby. Also, it's easier for infants to digest; "spitting up" is far more common in formula-fed babies, who often swallow air as well as formula.

Besides being nutritionally superior to animal milk and formulas, human milk helps the baby build up a resistance to diarrhea, rickets, anemia, allergies, polio, malaria, and a wide range of infections.[6] Infants who are breast-fed are also believed to have fewer orthodontic problems later in life.

". . . nursing and what happens around it seems to be the nuclear experience out of which develop all later feelings about oneself and other persons," according to Bruno Bettelheim. Many psychologists note that infants who are breast-fed seem more relaxed and contented, even as children.[7] An increasing body of evidence points to the conclusion that the psychological security provided by nursing has a permanent beneficial effect on the human personality.

Like a successful home birth, successful breast-feeding has to be worked at and planned for. If the mother wants to be able to provide a bountiful supply of milk, she ought to plan on eating more and sleeping more. She must also cultivate the ability to relax, to leave the household tasks undone, and to mentally take a vacation from everyday work while she nurses her baby. The psychological factor can't be minimized; if the woman becomes worried or uptight about anything, it will adversely affect her milk supply. Many a mother's attempts to breast-feed have gone on the rocks when she felt compelled to clean the house in preparation for an impending visit from her in-laws! Tension and fatigue are two of the biggest obstacles to having breast-feeding go smoothly. When the infant cries only an hour or two after she has nursed him, the frustrated mother can't be blamed for becoming discouraged.

To avoid these difficulties, one obstetrician tells his patients who plan to breast-feed that they should rest in bed during the first two weeks, except to care for themselves and their babies.[8] Besides rest, a lactating mother will probably need more sleep than usual. Some women need ten hours of sleep in order to avoid that tired, "all gone" feeling. Since the baby usually cries to be fed at night, a long nap during the daytime can help the mother get the sleep she needs.

Diet for the lactating woman can be about the same as during pregnancy, but she should drink extra milk and juices. One mother, when she is breast-feeding her baby, drinks a quart of milk each day, plus two quarts of water, tea, juices and soups. Every time a woman sits down to nurse her infant, drinking something helps to stimulate the flow of milk.

Many mothers discover that when they are nursing, they can eat twice as much as they normally do, but not gain weight. Food seems to taste twice as good. This is great, but be careful about chocolate, onions, cabbage, garlic, and brussels sprouts. Their flavors get into the milk and may upset the baby. Drugs and medicine can, too. A lactating woman took a laxative one night, to stimulate her sluggish bowels. The next morning, she complained that it hadn't worked.

"Oh yes it did," remarked her husband. "I just changed the baby's diapers!"

Breast-feeding a baby can require a lot of effort, but it's worth it. Besides benefiting the baby, it's good for the mother. The baby's sucking causes oxytocin to be released by the mother's pituitary gland, which stimulates her uterus to contract, helping it to return to its normal size. Nursing also creates "hormonal and psychological changes in the mother that promote maternal behavior."[9] Perhaps because of this, nursing mothers often seem to find their babies less of a chore to care for than mothers who bottle-feed.

For most women, breast-feeding delays ovulation. According to Dr. Allan Weingold, who heads the Maternal and Child Health Care Institute at New York Medical College's Metropolitan Hospital, a mother can become fertile again as early as three weeks after the birth of her baby. If she nurses the infant, however, ovulation may be delayed for about two years. Of course, nursing is not a foolproof method of birth control, as many couples have discovered!

Most books on childbirth advise couples to abstain from sexual relations until after the woman's postnatal checkup. Dr. Derek Llewellyn-Jones, the author of *Everywoman and Her Body,* does not think this six-week waiting period is strictly necessary. Sexual intercourse, he says, can safely be resumed after the disappearance of the lochia, or postpartum vaginal discharge. Some women who bear their children at home find their interest in sex returns quite quickly. This is probably because they experience much less perineal discomfort than women whose episiotomies are healing and whose muscles have been stretched on the delivery table.

A postnatal checkup, however, is a good idea, especially if

the mother has had her baby at home without medical supervision. During the six-week checkup, she can confirm that any superficial perineal tears have healed. The postnatal examination also affords her an opportunity to have a Pap test and a check for breast cancer. Information on family planning may be offered to her at this time, along with literature on exercises such as *Rapid Post Natal Figure Recovery*. This is an excellent booklet written by Constance Reed, a dance therapist, and published by Ortho Pharmaceuticals.

The baby should have a pediatric checkup when he is about six weeks old, too. It's a good opportunity to learn how much weight he has gained, and to get advice on starting him on solid foods. Baby-feeding recommendations seem to change almost as fast as clothing styles, but by the time they are about two months old, most babies enjoy small amounts of rice cereal and bananas or applesauce.

Infant immunizations can usually be started at the six-week checkup. Usually, the baby will receive an oral polio vaccine and a DPT shot, which will protect him from diptheria, whooping cough and tetanus. Be sure to get instructions on how to treat the baby's fever, as his reaction to the first immunization shot often seems to be more severe than later reactions.

By the time the infant is six weeks old, most parents are more than ready to help him settle into a regular schedule. While feeding on demand best meets the needs of a newborn infant, some kind of routine seems desirable if the two-month-old baby is to fit into his family rather than disrupt it. An unusual book that offers concrete advice in this area is *My First 300 Babies*, by Gladys West Hendrick, a California grandmother who has cared for almost 600 infants.

"Train up a child in the way he should go," says Proverbs, and *My First 300 Babies* explains why a well-ordered way of life should start from the cradle. Although Mrs. Hendrick's book stresses the importance of discipline and consistency, her love for her tiny charges comes through on every page. All her suggestions stem from a concern for the well-being of the child, not just for the sanity of his parents! It's a priceless antidote for the sometimes contradictory "guidelines" on child care which are currently offered to today's parents.

The baby's birth should be recorded within a few days after he is born. The easiest way to go about this is to call the County Office of Vital Statistics, which may also be listed in the telephone directory as Birth and Death Records. Ask them how to get a birth certificate. They will tell you where to go and what information to bring. If you take a few extra dollars to the Recorder's Office they will send you extra copies. It's a good idea to obtain several copies of the birth certificate. That way, they will be readily available when it's necessary to enter the child in school. The baby may also want to get a driver's license, a passport, or a marriage license some day. He will need his birth certificate for all of these.

When a baby is born in the hospital, the hospital usually registers his birth. Several weeks later, the parents must write to the county if they want copies of his birth certificate. But the parents of a home-born baby can attend to these details in person. Many a father takes justifiable pride in filling out his child's birth certificate; besides being the "father" on it, he may also be the "informant" and the "birth attendant." Testifying to the birth of his child can confirm the father's sense of parenthood. It underscores his self-confidence. After all, unlike most American men, he did not turn his wife over to the hospital for the birth, but accepted the responsibility himself. And now he has a healthy baby to show for it, plus a wife who has escaped the physical and psychological trauma of hospital childbirth.

Husbands who support their wives throughout pregnancy, childbirth, and lactation help to build strong family bonds. *Sexual Suicide* says the desire of men to identify and claim their children is one of the two cornerstones of civilization. (The other one is maternal feelings and practices.) By encouraging both of these impulses, childbirth at home may make far-reaching contributions toward a more human and civilized society.

"The very large issues of how men and women are to relate to each other and to their children, and of what kind of individuals we will be developing for the future, are . . . dependent upon the whole sequence of practices and policies surrounding pregnancy and gestation,"[10] according to Margaret Mead.

Another renowned anthropologist, Ashley Montagu, also recognizes the importance of childbirth customs.

> A hospital is a splendid place, but it is not, in my view, a place in which the most beautiful celebration in the history of a family, the welcoming of a new member into it, should occur. That event should be celebrated where it belongs, in the bosom of the family, in the home.[11]

NOTES

1. Lester Dessez Hazell, *Commonsense Childbirth* (New York: G.P. Putnam's Sons, 1969), p. 52.
2. Ibid., p. 164.
3. Raven Lang, *Birth Book* (Ben Lomond, California: Genesis Press, 1972.)
4. Hazell, op. cit., p. 165.
5. William D. Cochran, M.D., "Demand Feeding vs. Schedule Feeding," *Redbook*, March 1974, p. 154.
6. George Gilder, *Sexual Suicide* (New York: Quadrangle Books, 1973), p. 235.
7. "Doctor Favors Breast-Feeding," *The Sacramento Bee,* March 27, 1974, p. A10.
8. Joan Claire Gordon, Ed.D. and Ronald S. Gordon, Sc.D., "A Parents' Guide to Breast-Feeding, Part IV," *Marriage*, November 1974, p. 18.
9. George Gilder, op. cit., p. 235.
10. Boston Children's Medical Center, *Pregnancy, Birth and the Newborn Baby* (Boston: Boston Children's Medical Center, 1971), p. 59.
11. Robert A. Bradley, M.D., *Husband-Coached Childbirth* (New York: Harper & Row, 1965), x. (from the Preface by Ashley Montagu, Ph.D.)

OTHER SOURCES
(listed as they appear in text)

Boston Women's Health Book Collective, Inc., *Our Bodies, Ourselves* (New York: Simon & Schuster, 1973), p. 204.

"Human Milk Is Hailed As Resource," *The Sacramento Bee*, July 11, 1974, p. A14.

Bruno Bettelheim, M.D., *The Empty Fortress* (New York: The Free Press, 1967.)

Good Housekeeping, September 1970, p. 161.

Derek Llewellyn-Jones, M.D., *Everywoman and Her Body* (New York: Taplinger Publishing Company, 1971), p. 219.

Constance Reed, *Rapid Post Natal Figure Recovery* (Raritan, N.J.: Ortho Pharmaceutical Corporation, 1968.)

Gladys West Hendrick, *My First 300 Babies* (Pasadena, California: My First 300 Babies, 1964.)

AFTERWORD

MANAGEMENT OF THE COMPLICATIONS OF HOME DELIVERY: AN ANALYSIS OF RESULTS FROM THE SANTA CRUZ BIRTH CENTER, CALIFORNIA

by Lewis E. Mehl, M.D.
Departments of Family Practice and Psychiatry
University of Wisconsin Medical School
Madison, Wisconsin

and

Gail H. Peterson
School of Social Work
University of Wisconsin
Madison, Wisconsin

177

Editor's note:
The following chapter presents the results of a statistical analysis of almost 300 recent home deliveries. The figures were compliled at Stanford University in 1974. Although this is the type of information usually published in medical journals, we include it here because it confronts the question Americans ask most frequently about childbirth at hime—i.e., what happens if something goes wrong?

This is a report on the incidence and management of complications which occurred in a series of 287 home deliveries assisted by midwives from the Santa Cruz Birth Center in Santa Cruz, California. As far as we know, this is the first such statistical survey of recent American midwife-assisted home births. It provides data on the incidence with which certain complications occur at home, and describes how these complications were managed.

Ideally, every couple planning home delivery should be helped by a properly equipped physician and nurse-midwife team, backed up with means of rapid transport to a hospital setting. But, since few physicians are willing to become involved in home deliveries, this is usually not possible. In situations in which a physician is not present, birth attendants should have some idea of what kinds of complications may occur. Also, they should have some knowledge of how these complications have been handled by others.

Yet another important reason for studying home delivery outcomes is to address the question often posed by health-care providers regarding the safety of home delivery. For physicians to react rationally to the growing home birth trend, much more information must be available regarding maternal and infant complications and mortality-morbidity results. This is why we reviewed the records. Currently, as well, we are collecting statistics for 1,100 home births in the San Francisco Bay area, the results of which will soon be available.

From the Birth Center statistics it would appear paradoxically that home birth is safer than hospital birth. This statement should be qualified, since the *theoretical* risk is always higher in home delivery. However, the lessons learned from this study of home deliveries may be applicable to hospital births as well. That is, the more comfortable a woman is, the more relaxed the environment is, the more the woman is allowed to be surrounded by friends and relatives, the less pain-relieving medication and anesthesia is used, the more other positions for labor and delivery besides lying on the back are used, and the more the temptation to intervene in variants of normal labors is avoided, the safer and more desirable the hospital will become. However, some feel that the comfort and psychological safety of the home cannot be duplicated.

In general, it has been our impression that the kind of people choosing home delivery cover the range of people present in the community served, and that the reasons for electing home delivery are as varied as the ideologies about childbirth. (In Santa Cruz, the population tended to be more counter-culturally oriented than the population encountered in a physician-directed home delivery system.)

Raven Lang has described the formation and operation of the Santa Cruz Birth Center in *Birth Book*[1]. In brief, the Birth Center is composed of both lay and nurse midwives who have formed a collective to assist pregnant couples. They offer prenatal care, home delivery assistance, and postnatal followup, with an emphasis on self-responsibility of each pregnant couple. Midwives are trained by being apprenticed to more experienced midwives. They usually attend each home birth in groups of three: one to observe, and one to assist the more experienced midwife at the delivery.

Prenatal care involves the same number of visits as that recommended by physicians, with determination of blood pressure and urinary glucose, protein, pH, and ketones being done. Glucose is present in the urine in diabetes of pregnancy, while protein may be present in toxemia of pregnancy or in a bladder infection (cystitis) or kidney infection (pyelonephritis). Urinary tract infections such as these are associated with an increased incidence of premature delivery.

In addition, a careful analysis of the pregnant woman's diet is performed in early pregnancy; her diet is monitored until it meets standards of good nutrition. Each woman is requested to see a physician at least once, and preferably many times, during pregnancy for a Pap smear, gonorrhea culture, rubella titre, blood group and Rh typing, and a clinical estimate as to the size of her pelvis. She is also requested to obtain a hemoglobin and/or hematocrit determination at least twice, and preferably, three times during pregnancy so that if anemia is present, it can be treated with iron prior to delivery.

The complications studies were compiled from those women who were still planning a home delivery at the onset of labor. Of the original 322 women, only ten were screened out for medical reasons during pregnancy. (Five were eliminated because of a breech presentation, one for toxemia of pregnancy, one for diabetes of pregnancy, one for Rh incompatibility, and two for anemia.) Twenty-five other women chose to deliver in the hospital for psychosocial reasons, leaving a total of 287 women included in the study.

The average age of women giving birth was twenty-four, and

the average infant birth weight was 7½ lbs—66.8% of the women were having their first baby; their labors lasted an average of 17 hours—20.7% of the women were having their second baby; their labors lasted an average of 9½ hours—6.8% of the women were having their third baby; their labors lasted an average of 5 hours—2.3% of the women were having their fourth baby; their labors lasted an average of 6½ hours.

Of the 287 women who began labor at home, 45 of these required intervention at a hospital to complete their labor (15.7%). This number was lower in the physician-directed services, since some of the problems a lay midwife would have to take to the hospital could be handled by a doctor in the home. For example, a physician can administer buccal oxytocin (a hormone tablet sucked to stimulate the strength and duration of uterine contractions), and drugs such as methylergonovine to prevent excessive blood loss when it occurs after the birth.

In the remainder of this section, the complications encountered by the Birth Center will be discussed, in order to show how complications have been handled at home. (It is important to remember that 242 of the 287 births were completely normal deliveries and that only 45 women manifested the following complications for which 35 were taken to the hospital and 10 were able to manage at home. Some women had more than one complication.)

1. Meconium-stained amniotic fluid

Meconium in the waters imparts a light-golden to dark-green color to the amniotic fluid, according to whether it is old or new and according to the amount of meconium the infant is producing. Meconium can be a sign of distress, and when it occurs, the baby's heart rate should be listened to frequently. Some physicians feel that the presence of meconium in the waters is a certain sign of fetal distress, while others feel that without dropping of the fetal heart rate, meconium itself is not a problem. Regardless of this, it is very important to monitor the baby's heart rate if meconium occurs, and some parents will opt to go to the hospital at this point. The actual danger to the baby is that it will take the meconium into its mouth and breathe it into the lungs when the first breath is taken. If the meconium enters the lungs it causes a severe chemical irritation (meconium aspiration pneumonitis), which, in its most severe form, can prevent the baby from extracting sufficient oxygen from inspired air.

If the couple decides not to go to the hospital when meconium occurs, then most physicians would agree that the baby's mouth should be vigorously sucked out with a bulb syringe by the mother or another attendant after birth.

Six labors monitored by the Birth Center resulted in meconium waters (2.1%). All of the infants were born at home, and five of the resulting infants breathed spontaneously and had no difficulties. The sixth infant was a first baby born after a normal 6½ hour labor, weighing 5 lb. 10 oz. The birth was completely without incident with the exception of meconium one hour prior to delivery. The midwife was called late and arrived when the head was crowning, and no one had listened to the fetal heart rate during labor. The baby was born limp and did not breathe on its own for five minutes, although it received blood through the cord for one minute. Mouth-to-mouth resuscitation by the midwife was successful, and the infant was transported to a nearby hospital at which he proceeded to develop severe meconium aspiration pneumonitis and seizures from insufficient oxygen circulating to his brain (hypoxic seizures). During half of this time the baby required a respirator machine to do the work of breathing in order to maintain an oxygen level compatible with life. Three and a half years later, the infant had severe motor cerebral palsy but no mental retardation. The mother also had a viral illness during her first trimester of pregnancy, which may have contributed to this baby's condition, too. (However, the severity of the infant's symptoms might well have been lessened had his lungs been suctioned free of meconium immediately following his admission to the hospital.)

The incidence of meconium in hospital deliveries has been estimated at 10% for the total population.[2] The lower incidence of 2.1% in the home birth population occurs in other services besides the Santa Cruz group, so we believe this is a real phenomenon rather than the failure of lay midwives to report the occurrence of this complication. The reasons for a lower incidence of fetal distress in a home birth population are many, and will be discussed later.

2. Bleeding in labor

Bleeding during labor can be a symptom of potentially life-threatening complications for both mother and baby. The most dangerous causes are placenta previa, in which the placenta covers the opening of the cervix so that the baby cannot leave the uterus without going through the placenta, and abruptio placenta, in which the placenta separates early from the uterine wall and blood accumulates behind the placenta. Partial placenta previa means that part of the placenta covers the opening of the cervix, and partial abruptio placenta means that only a portion of the placenta has separated from the uterus. In a complete abruptio placenta the baby cannot survive long because its source of blood and oxygen has been severed, although in a partial abruptio placenta, even though the amount of oxygen and blood the baby is receiving may have diminished, the baby still receives enough blood to maintain life—at least for the time being.

The signs of abruptio placenta include the signs of shock in the mother (a weak, thready pulse, cool, pale skin, sweating, and a feeling of weakness and impending doom), enlargement of the uterus from the blood collecting inside, and a decline of the fetal heart rate as less blood reaches the infant through the placenta. Placenta previa is usually diagnosed by a vaginal exam in the hospital with a speculum. If it is present, then bleeding will usually become intense after such a vaginal exam, and a Caesarean section must be done immediately. If bleeding occurs during labor the woman should be taken to the hospital, unless a physician is in the home to evaluate the situation. For more information see references[3] and [4].

In the Birth Center statistics four women (1.4%) had blood-tinged amniotic fluid during labor, probably as a result of small cervical blood vessels breaking during dilation. This bleeding stopped almost immediately after it started, and all labors were normal at home.

3. Toxemia of pregnancy

Toxemia of pregnancy is a complication usually uncovered during prenatal care, and, as Dr. Tom Brewer[5] has shown, it is intimately related to deficient protein intake and other nutritional deficiencies. The symptoms include high blood pressure, and edema (swelling of the fingers and legs). Often there is a very large weight gain which is associated with body retention of fluid. (Some edema *without* hypertension is normal in pregnancy, and should not be confused with toxemia—in which high blood pressure is always present.) Nutritional counseling and education can help prevent many cases of toxemia, but occasionally the first indications of toxemia may occur during labor with an elevated blood pressure. For this reason, it is important to measure the blood pressure at regular intervals during labor. The blood pressure levels at which a woman shuold be taken to the hospital are controversial, but most would agree that anyone with a blood pressure of 140/100 during labor should be in the hospital. Symptoms of high blood pressure include headaches, nosebleeds, blurred vision, and dizziness; although all of these symptoms can come from other causes.

At the Birth Center on a prenatal care day, one woman arrived in early labor. She had had no prenatal care and expected to deliver at the Birth Center. She was 20 years old, having her first child, and was convinced by the Birth Center midwives to go to the hospital. Her blood pressure at the Birth Center was 160/120—(normal is 120/80)—and at the hospital her blood pressure continued to increase; a Caesarean section was done four hours later. Both she and her baby did well afterwards. One other woman had a high blood pressure during labor (to 140/95) but she refused to go to the hospital. She had a normal home delivery, her high blood pressure subsiding immediately after birth.

4. Cervical edema

Swelling of the cervix usually occurs when a woman pushes before the cervix is fully dilated. When the infant's head pushes against the cervix, it becomes very thickened (edematous). This complication can be prevented by a vaginal exam before a woman begins to push, to determine if there is any cervix remaining. Sometimes women can successfully push a baby through the cervix even though a portion of it (called a lip) remains; if the woman has an overwhelming desire to push, this may be successful.

Mild to moderate cervical edema is usually managed by the woman blowing through her contractions until the cervix has vanished, and then she begins to push. Often changing the mother's position so that the portion of the cervix which remains present is toward the ground is helpful; gravity will then help this lip to disappear. Thus if a portion of the cervix remains toward the front, and the woman has been laboring lying on her back, she might then change to the knee-chest position. Sometimes the cervix can also be eased over the baby's head during a contraction if it's particularly difficult for it to finish dilating, but this should only be done by someone experienced with this technique.

Cervical edema occurred once (0.35%) in the Birth Center statistics in a 23-year-old woman having her first child. She had begun to push at 6 cm. cervical dilatation. (Complete dilatation is 10 centimeters). The woman was taken to the hospital where 200 milligrams of secobarbital were given, which allowed her to relax. The cervix then finished dilating. The baby was born vaginally six hours after arriving at the hospital and did not breathe right away at birth, but required three minutes of resuscitation.

5. Neonatal jaundice

Mild jaundice (hyperbilirubinemia) is common in newborns and is manifested as yellowing of the skin and eyes between the second and the fifth days of life. It's caused by a delay in the ability of the newborn's liver to deal with bilirubin, a product of the breakdown of hemoglobin (the oxygen-carrying molecule of the blood) from used-up red blood cells. Abnormal jaundice is jaundice occurring prior to the second day of life or after the fifth day of life, or jaundice between the second and fifth day that's particularly severe. If the parents are worried about the baby's yellowness, a physician should be consulted. If the color is particularly worrisome, he or she might recommend that a blood bilirubin level be determined; (blood bilirubin levels over 20 milligrams per 100 cc's of blood can cause brain damage.) Causes of abnormal jaundice include infection, blood group incompatibility, structural abnormality in the liver, and many other possibilities. Further information can be found in references 2 and 6–8.

Therapy of abnormally high jaundice consists of placing the

infant under high intensity lights to lower the blood bilirubin concentration. Unfortunately, this therapy often separates mother and infant, since phototherapy is usually continuous until the bilirubin is within safe limits. This may also have an adverse psychological effect on the infant because of sensory deprivation; he must be blindfolded to prevent damage to the eyes. Recently, however, Zachman[9] has shown that phototherapy is just as effective when it is administered every *other* day, thus decreasing the psychosocial complications.

Nine Birth Center babies required phototherapy for excessive jaundice (3.15%). In one of the cases, a physician helped the mother devise a home phototherapy unit so that the baby would not have to be hospitalized. The other eight infants were hospitalized for varying periods of time for phototherapy. The cause of jaundice was never determined in any of the nine babies, and jaundice resolved in all.

6. Stillbirth

Stillbirth was noted once in the Birth Center statistics (0.35%). For no determinable reason, the infant died four weeks prior to the due date, and the mother delivered a slightly decomposed (autolyzed) infant at that time. Vigorous mouth-to-mouth resuscitation was performed anyway by an attendant who could not accept that the infant had died. The autopsy report revealed autolysis (decomposition caused by the release of destructive enzymes from dead cells), maceration (the external evidence of autolysis such as peeling of the skin), and some air in the lungs —presumably secondary to the mouth-to-mouth resuscitory efforts. This unfortunate complication is detectable during prenatal care, of course, by a sudden absence of fetal heart sounds. It is important that a dead fetus be delivered relatively soon to prevent additional medical complications in the mother. (See reference 3).

7. Abnormal presentation

a. Posterior labor is the most common abnormal presentation occurring at home; it occurred 30 times in the Birth Center group. A posterior labor occurs when the baby's face is looking in the direction of the mother's belly. It is a more difficult labor because the infant's head is not in the right position to mold to the shape of the birth canal. Many posterior babies often turn to anterior (looking toward the mother's back) after causing some degree of back discomfort and lengthening the labor. This occurred in fifteen of the women who had posterior labors, and they were able to remain at home for normal deliveries.

The other half of the thirty women were taken to the hospital after having long labors without much progress. All the women were given the hormone oxytocin (the natural substance which initiates and maintains labor in women). This made their contractions stronger and longer, and twelve went on to have normal vaginal deliveries. In ten of these twelve, with the increased strength of uterine contractions, the babies turned from the posterior to the normal anterior position, and in the other two labors the babies remained posterior and were delivered "sunny side up." Three of the women showed no progress in labor even after being given oxytocin, and an X ray in each case showed that the babies' heads were too large to fit through the mothers' birth canals (cephalopelvic disproportion), so Caesarean deliveries were performed. Posterior labors averaged 2.4 times longer than normal anterior labors.

  b. Brow presentation is a rare position in which the brow of the face is the lowest part of the baby in the birth canal, the part which dilates the cervix by pushing against it and leads the baby's descent into the birth canal. Normally the top of the head, or crown, is the lowest part in the birth canal, and indeed, the baby's skull bones are designed so that when this part is acting as the battering ram, the skull bones will mold well to fit the configuration of the birth canal. Brow presentation occurs 0.096% of the time.[10] The one time (0.35%) it occurred in the Birth Center deliveries was in a labor taken to the hospital when the mother was unable to push the baby out. The infant was on the perineum near the vaginal opening, but was wedged in place. After a large episiotomy, it was delivered by low forceps. (Low refers to the baby's position in the birth canal; in a mid-forceps delivery, the baby is about midway between cervix and vaginal opening when the forceps are applied to its head. In a high forceps delivery, the baby has made virtually no descent into the birth canal.)

  Whenever brow presentation occurs, it should be transported to the hospital immediately unless an easy delivery is imminent, or a physician is present to evaluate the situation. For more information, see references 3, 10 and 11.

  c. Breech presentation (butt first instead of head first) occurred in five women who were not included in these statistics since the breech was diagnosed prenatally and they were referred to the hospital prior to the onset of labor. Breech deliveries can be very dangerous if the head is larger than the pelvic girdle. Some physicians with oxygen and resuscitator equipment available will deliver breech babies at home, but only if there is at least one-half centimeter on either side of the baby's head when the largest head diameter is compared to the smallest diameter of the mother's birth canal. Other doctors will not deliver breech at home regardless of the circumstances. Some obstetricians have gone so far as to recommend Caesarean section of all first-baby breeches, although this seems an extremist position. One point virtually everyone will agree with is that a breech delivery should never be attempted at home without the presence of a physician experienced in delivering breeches, and without the presence of oxygen and resuscitation equipment. For more information see references 3, 12–14, and 27.

d. *Twins* did not occur in this series from the Birth Center, but the same considerations about breech delivery at home apply to twin delivery at home. For more information on delivery technique see reference 3.

8. Prematurity

An infant weighing less than 2500 grams at birth (about 5½ lbs.) is defined as premature. Any labor which takes place more than two to three weeks prior to the due date should be taken to the hospital, unless a physician has performed an ultrasound examination to determine the size of the infant and has determined that the infant is full-term. Premature infants usually develop a lung disease called respiratory distress syndrome or hyaline membrane disease. This is characterized by an inability of the infant to extract sufficient oxygen from the air breathed in. It occurs because of a lack of a molecule called a surfactant which lines the lung and keeps the small airways in the lung expanded. Without this molecule the small airways would collapse each time a person exhales; this is essentially what happens in premature infants.

The signs of this respiratory disease in infants include a blue color (cyanosis), flaring or enlargement of the nostrils with each breath, a very rapid rate of breathing, a grunting noise with each breath, and a caving in of the sternum in the middle of the chest with each breath (retractions). For more information on this see references 2, 6, and 15–18. Other problems frequently manifested by premature infants include an inability to suck strongly, hypoglycemia, and an inability to maintain body temperature. Maternal cigarette smoking has been associated with prematurity,[19] as has maternal urinary tract infection during pregnancy and poor nutrition.

Eight Birth Center babies were premature (2.8%). Six of the babies were born in a hospital and two were born at home. One of the infants born at home weighed 4 lbs. 10 oz., developed mild lung disease and was hospitalized. The other home-born infant weighed 5 lbs. and did well at home. Another nursing mother helped the mother nurse the baby until her milk came in, in order to prevent hypoglycemia. (Infants weighing less than 5 lb. 10 oz. or more than 8 lb. 12 oz. are considered more susceptible to hypoglycemia following birth.) Of the premature babies born in the hospital, one had severe lung disease as a result of being born two months early, three had mild disease, and two had no disease.

9. Prolonged labor

Friedman[20-22] has divided the first stage of labor into two parts: the latent phase (early labor) and the active phase (active or hard labor). Early labor is characterized by weak, irregularly spaced contractions with slow dilatation on the cervix. Suddenly the contractions become harder, more regular, and dilatation of the cervix proceeds much more rapidly. This is the active phase, which usually begins at about four centimeters of cervical dilatation. A prolonged first stage of labor in itself is not necessarily harmful to the infant as long as some progress is being made. Thus, it is not the *speed* of progress but rather the *presence* of progress (progressive cervical dilatation) which is important.* Causes of a prolonged first stage include uterine inertia, in which the contractions are weak and ineffectual, and dysfunctional labor, in which the contractions seem strong, but are not effectual. Dysfunctional labor also includes labor which goes on for a long time with irregular contractions which don't become regular.

Friedman has stated that such prolonged labors "do not contribute in any detectable way to infant mortality." In the same way, a prolonged second stage (usually defined as longer than two hours) in which there remains slow descent of the head in the birth canal offers no increase in risks to the baby born vaginally. Long second stages are dangerous only to the extent that they are accompanied by the use of forceps in delivery.[24] "Thus it would seem that the protraction pattern (slow labor) does not of itself contribute to the poor results sometimes encountered, but rather they are obtained from the potentially traumatic operative procedures used for delivery (forceps delivery)."

If the cervix actually stops dilating in active labor (called arrest of dilatation by Friedman) or if the baby actually stops descending in the birth canal during the pushing stage (called arrest of descent by Friedman), then a situation of inherent danger to the infant results, but just as in the non-dangerous slowing of labor, the use of forceps markedly increases the risk to the baby. Friedman has found that low forceps deliveries increase infant mortality 1.9 times when used in normal deliveries, 12 times after long active labors, and 1.5 times when the baby fails to be pushed out of the birth canal. Mid-forceps delivery increases infant mortality 7.2 times in normal deliveries, 10.8 times after long early labors, 28.5 times after long active labors, and 2.4 times if the baby fails to be pushed down the birth canal. (These numbers compare to the same delivery accomplished without the use of any forceps.)

When forceps were not used, infant death rate was not increased over normal deliveries, in deliveries with a long early labor, a long active labor, or a long pushing stage. When labor had actually stopped, however, the infant death rate increased 16 times—even when forceps were not used. These results were obtained from

---

* Although it is sometimes very difficult to differentiate between very slow progress and a lack of progress. This often requires several highly-trained observers and a trial of oxytocin.

3000 deliveries, the majority of them *not* in distressed infants. (For more information see reference 24.)

The point at which a long labor should be taken to the hospital is very difficult to decide, then, regardless of the above considerations Friedman has made, since attendants of home deliveries have varying levels of capability to assess the progress of labor. Such a decision will of course depend on the birth attendants' competence and confidence, the mother's intuition and energy reserve, and the condition of the baby. Most would agree that absolute indications in a long labor would be maternal exhaustion, attendant confusion, a dropping of the fetal heart rate, or an intuition from the mother that something is wrong.

In the Birth Center statistics, 20 women had a prolonged first stage (longer than 24 hours). The average length of labor in these women was 40 hours, and the range was 25 to 72 hours. Two Caesarean deliveries were performed because of a complete cessation of cervical dilatation in active labor. In both cases, the babies were too large to fit through the mother's pelvis.

Fifteen other women went to the hospital and received oxytocin to increase the strength of their uterine contractions, since the contractions seemed weak and ineffectual (uterine inertia). In all but two of the women, this had occurred in active labor. The other two women had never gone beyond early labor. Three of these women had forceps deliveries. The average woman went to the hospital after laboring at home for 28 hours and with an average cervical dilatation of seven centimeters.

Of the three women who labored at home, one had a 72 hour labor, but with only ten hours of active labor. She was a 22-year-old woman having her first child, and at one point, labor stopped —enabling her to sleep for eight hours. Labor resumed when she awoke; her baby was in excellent condition at birth. Another home delivery was entirely normal except for a 26 hour first stage. The final home birth of this group occurred in a 31-year-old woman having her first child, assisted by a friend who was a physician. She had a 39 hour first stage and was given oxytocin by mouth at home to stimulate her uterus, because of weak, ineffectual contractions. The baby was born in excellent condition and there was moderate bleeding after the birth of the placenta. The midwife present administered a concentrated herbal tea, blue cohosh, which she believed to be helpful in contracting the uterus; bleeding ceased shortly thereafter.

Prolonged second stage is usually diagnosed when pushing requires longer than two hours. Eight women met this criterion. The range in length was from two hours, two minutes to six hours. Half of the women had normal deliveries at home and the other half went to the hospital. Three of these had forceps deliveries, and one was given oxytocin to stimulate her contractions, after which she gave birth spontaneously.

10. Retained placenta

This condition occurred in three women who were taken to the hospital where their placentas were manually removed.

11. Prolonged rupture of membranes

When the bag of waters is broken longer than 24 hours prior to delivery, the risk of intra-uterine infection increases with the length of time that the waters are broken. There has been some controversy regarding whether infant infection is certain after the waters are broken for more than 24 hours. In a study of 6,269 deliveries from Kaiser Hospital, Los Angeles, Sachs and Baker[23] showed that the incidence of infection was not increased in full-term babies unless the mother showed signs of infection such as fever or foul-smelling waters. Similar findings were reported from seven U.S.Navy Hospitals in 13,383 deliveries.[24]

Russell and Anderson[25] have disagreed with these findings after studying 31,865 deliveries in Los Angeles County Hospital, a large county hospital serving a primarily lower socioeconomic, largely indigent population. Thus hygiene and socioeconomic status (which often reflects nutritional status) are also important. Webb[26] has reported 54 preventable maternal deaths from prolonged broken waters, so that it is probably important to induce labor if there are no indications that active labor has begun 24 hours after the waters have broken.

Seven women in the Birth Center group manifested this problem and three went to the hospital for induction of labor. Three had already gone to the hospital because of a prolonged first stage. One baby was delivered at home and did well; the other six infants were in excellent condition, also.

12. Perineal tears requiring repair

Perineal tears occurred in 55 women. Two women had tears into the rectum and four had tears into the sphincter muscle around the rectum. Fourteen women were sutured at home, forty went to the hospital for stitches, and one refused to be sutured, with a poor result. When an experienced midwife was involved in the delivery, only 6% of the women tore enough to require repair; when fathers or inexperienced midwives caught babies, this number increased to 17%. Factors preventing perineal tearing have been outlined by Raven Lang[1] and include good perineal massage before birth and while the baby is crowning, a slow, well-controlled delivery of the head and shoulders, and prenatal perineal massage. (When perineal massage is performed during labor, sterile gloves should be worn to guard against the possibility of infection.

13. Uterine Infections

Infections in the uterus occurred in five women after birth (1.8%). One was hospitalized for two days; the others were

treated as outpatients with antibiotics. This rate is similar to that
of the hospital.

14. Breathing problems

Problems in breathing occurred in nine infants. Five of these
were premature and have already been mentioned, as was one
meconium-stained infant, and one infant born after the mother
sustained cervical edema. Two other babies required five minutes of stimulation to achieve a good breathing pattern but did
not need mouth-to-mouth resuscitation. Both are normal children now, two and three years old.

15. Postpartum hemorrhage

Heavy bleeding occurred in three women. All had normal
home births and delivered healthy infants at home. Two of the
three could have been prevented if drugs to control hemorrhage
(oxytocin and methylergonovine) had been available to be administered at home when bleeding began. The first hemorrhage
occurred in a 21-year-old woman having her first baby. She
began bleeding moderately following the birth of the placenta.
Efforts to stimulate her uterus to contract and thereby stop the
bleeding were in vain, so she was transported in a head-down
position to a hospital by car within eight minutes after birth.
Upon arrival she had lost one liter of blood (about a quart) and
had a blood pressure of 60/30 (within shock levels) for two hours
after arrival. She was given methylergonovine to stop the bleeding and hemorrhage ceased after the second dose of this drug,
nineteen minutes after delivery. Four hours later she left the
emergency room.

The second woman retained a piece of placenta and was immediately taken to the hospital. She arrived within 15 minutes
and had lost about two liters (quarts) of blood. Upon arrival, the
placenta remaining in her uterus was manually removed and she
was given a pint of blood. Her blood pressure remained at 80/40
for eight hours and she was in the hospital for two days, recover-
ing from the mild shock she had sustained; she left the hospital in
good condition.

The third hemorrhage occurred in a 25-year-old woman having her first child; she began a slow, persistent bleeding after
birth. She was taken to the hospital where she continued to bleed,
despite the administration of oxytocin and methylergonovine.
Finally she was given a pint of whole blood, after which the
bleeding stopped. She had a history of bleeding for three days
after having a tooth pulled on two separate occasions, and had
refused to have a hospital delivery even though it had been
strongly recommended to her.(That the whole blood stopped her
bleeding indicated that she probably had a defect in her ability to
clot blood.)

16. Cervical tearing

Cervical tearing occurred three times. Two occurred in women who delivered in the hospital because of prolonged first stages and had mid-forceps deliveries. The other cervical tear occurred in a 25-year-old woman having a normal first baby at home; there were no problems and the tear was repaired in the hospital. The danger of cervical tearing is that the tear might extend into the uterus and cause hemorrhage. This did not occur in these three women.

After reading about the various complications, it is important to remember that 84% of the home deliveries were entirely normal. Of course, when planning a home delivery it's a good idea to keep in mind that the birth may have complications. Probably the woman's own intuition about her pending birth is the best indicator for where she should deliver—(assuming that no complications were uncovered during prenatal care).

Of the 287 births studied, 3.5% were delivered by Caesarean section, and 1.0% were forceps deliveries. (In Santa Cruz County during the same time period, 8.4% births were Caesarean deliveries.)

There are many reasons which might explain the good results obtained by the Birth Center women. One explanation could be that the midwives failed to report complications which occurred, but we believe this false, since other home birth services we are currently studying have similar low incidences of complications. Perhaps because of the presence of physicians, some are even lower than the Birth Center's. A major factor seems to be the avoidance of pain-relieving medication and anesthesia. Many studies have commented upon the association of pain-relieving drugs and anesthesia with more infant breathing problems and greater numbers of infants requiring resuscitation.[28-34]

Another important influence on the statistics may have been the position assumed by women in labor. Forty-two percent of the mothers delivered their babies at home in positions other than on the back and Lamaze positions. In hospitals women are usually on their backs during labor and delivery even though many studies have shown that, in this position, the weight of the baby and the enlarged uterus can compress the aorta; this decreases the amount of blood flowing to the uterus and hence through the placenta to the baby[35-37]. Goodlin has suggested that no woman should labor lying on her back for this reason[36].

An interesting note relating to the meconium stained infants in this series is that three were born after women labored on their backs, and three after labors in the Lamaze position (back at a 45 degree angle). Although 33.9% of the mothers delivered their babies in the hands and knees position, none of their infants had meconium staining. Compression of the aorta is not possible in the hands and knees position. It would be interesting to further study the effect of maternal position in labor in relation to the incidence of meconium appearing in the waters, to determine if this can be prevented by laboring in positions which do not compress the aorta.

Another factor contributing to the good outcomes in birth at home may be absence of fear. Kelly[38] has shown that fear decreases blood flow to the uterus and thus to the baby. Fear may be much lower in a comfortable home environment with loving and friendly attendants than in the more sterile and less friendly environment of the hospital. Conversely, if a woman had more fear of giving birth in the home than in the hospital, then there may be more risk for her to deliver at home.

The disturbance of labor which often occurs in a hospital may also be an important factor, since Newton[30] has shown that in mice whose labors are environmentally disturbed, labors may be as much as 72% longer and there may be as many as 54% more dead pups. Home environments are probably more conducive toward a relaxed labor than the relatively strange hospital environment. For a detailed consideration of hospital-caused disturbances see reference 40.

Home birth, then, would seem to be a safe reality. This is especially true when the laboring woman has shown no abnormalities during prenatal care, and when her delivery is attended by trained individuals. The good results obtained in home births ought to encourage the development of well-equipped American home delivery services, as well as improvement in hospital procedures to make hospital birth more "home-like."

Many have pointed out that as yet, home births constitute a very tiny minority of all American births. This is partly due to the lack of available statistics on them. We hope that this report of the good results of home deliveries will encourage the collection of more statistics about them.

REFERENCES
(listed as they appear in text)

1. Lang, Raven, *Birth Book,* Ben Lomond, California: Genesis Press, 1972.
2. Klaus, M. and A. Farnoff, ed., *Care of the High Risk Neonate,* W.B. Saunders and Co., Toronto, 1973.
3. Friedman, E.A., *Textbook of Obstetrics,* W.B. Saunders and Co., Toronto, 1974.
4. Hubbard, B.M. and T.N.A. Jeffcoate, "Abru   '   ¬nta," *Obstetrics and Gynecology* 27: 155-167, 1966.
5. Brewer, T., *Nutritional Basis of Pregnancy,* International Childbirth Education Association Supply House, Seattle, Washington, 1974.
6. Barnett, P., ed., *Pediatrics,* McGraw-Hill, New York, N.Y., 1974, 14th edition.
7. Johnson, J.D., "Neonatal non-hemolytic jaundice," *New England Journal of Medicine* 292: 194-197, 1975.
8. Hill, R.M., J.H. Kennel, and A.C. Barnes, "Vitamin K administration and neonatal hyperbilirubinemia of unknown etiology," *American Journal of Obstetrics and Gynecology* 82: 320-324, 1961.
9. Zachman, R.D., "Alternate phototherapy in neonatal hyperbilirubinemia," *Biology of the Neonate 25:* 283-288, 1974.
10. Mostar, S., E. Akaltin, and C. Babuna, "Deflexion attitudes: median vertex, persistent brow, and face presentations," *Obstetrics and Gynecology 28:* 49-56, 1966.
11. Cucco, U.P., "Face presentation," *American Journal of Obstetrics and Gynecology 94:* 1085-1097, 1966.
12. Patterson, S.P., R.C. Mulliniks, P.C. Shreier, "Breech presentation in the primigravida," *American Journal of Obstetrics and Gynecology 98:* 405-410, 1967.
13. Zatuchni, G.I. and G.J. Andros, "Prognostic index for vaginal delivery in breech presentation at term," *American Journal of Obstetrics and Gynecology 93:* 237-242, 1965.
14. Morley, G.W., "Breech presentation—a 15 year review," *Obstetrics and Gynecology, 30:* 745-751, 1967.
15. Clements, J.A., et al., "Assessment of the risk of the respiratory-distress syndrome by a rapid test for surfactant in amniotic fluid," *New England Journal of Medicine 286:* 1077-1081, 1972.
16. Johnson, J.D., Malachowski, N.C., Grobstein, R., Welsh, D., Daily, W.J.R., and P. Sunshine, "Prognosis of children surviving with the aid of mechanical ventilations in the newborn period," *Journal of Pediatrics 84:* 272-276, 1974.

17. Harrod, J.R., P.O. L'Heureux, O.D. Wangenstein, and C.E. Hunt, "Long-term follow-up of severe respiratory distress syndrome treated with IPPB," *Journal of Pediatrics 84:* 277-286, 1974.

18. Chernick, V., "Hyaline-membrane disease—therapy with constant-distending pressure," *New England Journal of Medicine 289:* 302-305, 1973.

19. Peterson, W.F., K.N. Morese, and D.F. Kaltreider, "Smoking and Prematurity: A preliminary report based on study of 7,740 Caucasians," *Obstetrics and Gynecology* 775-779, 1965.

20. Friedman, E.A., "Patterns of labor as indicators of risk," *Clinical Obstetrics and Gynecology,* Summer, 1974.

21. Friedman, E.A. and M.R. Sachtleben, "Dysfunctional labor v. Therapeutic trial of oxytocin in secondary arrest," *Obstetrics and Gynecology 21:* 13-21, 1963.

22. Friedman, E.A., "The functional division of labor," *American Journal of Obstetrics and Gynecology 109:* 274-279, 1971.

23. Sachs, M. and T.H. Baker, "Spontaneous premature rupture of the membranes: a prospective study," *American Journal of Obstetrics and Gynecology 97:* 888-893, 1967.

24. Lebherz, T.B., C.R. Boyce, J.W. Hustos, "Premature rupture of the membranes: A statistical study from 7 U.S. Navy hospitals," *American Journal of Obstetrics and Gynecology 81:* 658-665, 1961.

25. Russell, K.P. and G.V. Anderson, "The aggressive management of ruptured membranes," *American Journal of Obstetrics and Gynecology 83:* 930-937, 1962.

26. Webb, G.A., "Maternal death associated with premature rupture of the membranes: An analysis of 54 cases," *American Journal of Obstetrics and Gynecology 98:* 594-601, 1967.

27. Tank, E.S., R. Davis, J.F. Holt, G.W. Morley, "Mechanisms of trauma during breech delivery," *Obstetrics and Gynecology 38:* 761-767, 1971.

28. Bowes, W. et al., "The effects of obstetrical medication on fetus and infant," *Monographs of the Society for Research on Child Development,* Vol. 35, No. 137, June 1970.

29. Brazelton, T.B., "Effect of maternal medication on the neonate and his behavior," *Journal of Pediatrics 58:* 513-518, May 1961.

30. Richards, M., and J. Bernal, "Effects of obstetric medication on mother-infant interaction and infant development," *Third International Congress of Psychosomatic Medicine in Obstetrics and Gynecology,* London, April 1971.

31. Baker, J., "The effects of drugs on the fetus," *Pharmacological Reviews 12:* 37-90, 1960.

32. Werboff, J. and R. Kesner, "Learning deficits of offspring after administration of tranquilizing drugs to the mother," *Nature 197:* 106-107, September 1963.

33. James, L.S., "The effects of pain relief for labor and delivery on the fetus and newborn," *Anesthesiology 21:* 405-430, April 1960.

34. Vasecky, A., "Fetal bradycardia after paracervical block," *Obstetrics and Gynecology 38:* 500-512, June 1971.
35. Blankfield, A., "The optimum position for childbirth," *Medical Journal of Australia 2:* 666-668, June 1965.
36. Goodlin, R.C., "Importance of the lateral position during labor," *Obstetrics and Gynecology 37:* 698-702, July 1971.
37. Humphey, M., Haenslow, D., Morgan, S., and Wood, C., "The influence of maternal position at birth on the fetus," *Journal of Obstetrics and Gynecology of the British Commonwealth 80:* 1075-1080, December 1973.
38. Kelly, J., "Effect of fear upon uterine mobility," *American Journal of Obstetrics and Gynecology 83:* 576-581, June 1962.
39. Newton, N., "The effects of disturbance on labor," *American Journal of Obstetrics and Gynecology 101:* 1096-1102, September 1968.
40. Shaw, N., *Forced Labor: Maternity Care in the United States*, Elmsford, New York: Pergamon Press, Inc., 1974.

BIBLIOGRAPHY

BOOKS:

Alk, Madelin, ed. *The Expectant Mother—a Redbook Documentary,* New York: Trident Press, 1967.

Anonymous, M.D. *Confessions of a Gynecologist.* Garden City, New York: Doubleday & Co., Inc., 1972.

Apgar, Virginia, M.D., and Joan Beck. *Is My Baby All Right?* New York: Trident Press, 1972.

Bean, Constance A. *Methods of Childbirth.* Garden City, New York: Doubleday & Co., Inc., 1972.

Bettelheim, Bruno, M.D. *The Empty Fortress—Infantile Autism and the Birth of the Self.* New York: The Free Press, 1967.

Bing, Elisabeth D., ed. *The Adventure of Birth.* New York: Simon & Schuster, 1970.

Bing, Elisabeth. *Six Practical Lessons for an Easier Childbirth.* New York: Grosset & Dunlap, 1967.

Bird, Caroline. *Born Female.* New York: David McKay, 1970.

Bonstein, Isidore, M.D. *Psychoprophylactic Preparation for Painless Childbirth.* London: Morrison & Gibb, Ltd., 1958.

Boston Children's Medical Center. *Pregnancy, Birth and the Newborn Baby.* Boston: Boston Children's Medical Center, 1971.

Boston Women's Health Book Collective, Inc. *Our Bodies, Ourselves.* New York: Simon & Schuster, 1973.

Bradley, Robert A., M.D. *Husband-Coached Childbirth.* New York: Harper & Row, 1965, 1974.

Brewer, Thomas A., M.D. *If You Are Pregnant and Want Your Child . . .* Berkeley, California: Student Research Facility, (N.D.)

Brewer, Thomas A., M.D. *Metabolic Toxemia of Late Pregnancy.* Springfield, Illinois: Charles C. Thomas, 1966.

Brown, Janet, et al. *Two Births.* New York: Random House, and Berkeley, California: The Bookworks, 1972.

Buxton, C. Lee, M.D. *A Study of Psychophysical Methods for Relief of Childbirth Pain.* Philadelphia: W.B. Saunders Co., 1962.

Carter, Patricia Cloyd. *Come Gently, Sweet Lucina.* Titusville, Florida: Patricia Cloyd Carter, 1957.

Chabon, Irwin, M.D. *Awake and Aware.* New York: Delacorte Press, 1966.

Cherry, Sheldon H., M.D. *Understanding Pregnancy and Childbirth.* Indianapolis: Bobbs-Merrill, 1973.

Cohen, Allen. *Childbirth Is Ecstasy.* San Francisco: Aquarius Publishing Company, 1971.

Colman, Arthur and Libby. *Pregnancy: The Psychological Experience.* New York: Herder & Herder, 1971.

Dalton, Katherina, M.D. *The Menstrual Cycle.* New York: Pantheon Books, 1969.

Davis, Adelle. *Let's Have Healthy Children.* New York: Harcourt Brace Jovanovich, 1972.

Dick-Read, Grantly, M.D. *Childbirth Without Fear.* New York: Harper & Row, 1944, 1959.

Eastman, Nicholson J., M.D. and Keith P. Russell, M.D. *Expectant Motherhood.* Boston: Little, Brown & Co., 1970.

Eloesser, Leo, Edith J. Galt, and Isabel Hemingway, *Pregnancy, Childbirth and the Newborn: A Manual for Rural Midwives.* Mexico City: Instituto Indigenista Interamericano, 1959.

Ewy, Donna, and Rodger. *Preparation for Childbirth—A Lamaze Guide.* Boulder, Colorado: Pruett Publishing Co., 1970.

Flanagan, Geraldine Lux. *The First Nine Months of Life.* New York: Simon & Schuster, 1962.

Fleury, P.M. *Maternity Care—Mothers' Experiences of Childbirth.* London: George Allen & Unwin Ltd., 1967.

Frankfort, Ellen. *Vaginal Politics.* New York: Quadrangle Books, 1972.

Gilder, George F. *Sexual Suicide.* New York: Quadrangle Books, 1973.

Goodrich, Frederick W., M.D. *Preparing for Childbirth.* Englewood, N.J.: Prentice-Hall, Inc., 1966.

Green, George Herbert, M.D. *Introduction to Obstetrics.* Christchurch, N.Z.: E.M. Peryer Ltd., 1966.

Greer, Germaine. *The Female Eunuch.* New York: McGraw-Hill Book Co., 1970.

Guttmacher, Alan F., M.D. *Pregnancy, Birth and Family Planning.* New York: The Viking Press, 1973.

Hazell, Lester Dessez. *Commonsense Childbirth.* New York: G.P. Putnam's Sons, 1969.

Heardman, Helen. *A Way to Natural Childbirth.* Edinburgh: F. & S. Livingstone, 1970.

Hendrick, Gladys West. *My First 300 Babies.* Pasadena, California: My First 300 Babies, 1964.

Karlins, Marvin, and Lewis M. Andrews. *Biofeedback.* New York: Warner Books, Inc., 1973.

Karmel, Marjorie. *Thank You, Dr. Lamaze.* Philadelphia: J.B. Lippincott, 1959.

Kitzinger, Sheila. *The Experience of Childbirth.* New York: Taplinger Publishing Co., 1962.

Lamaze, Fernand, M.D. *Painless Childbirth.* New York: Henry Regnery Co., 1970.

Lang, Raven. *Birth Book.* Ben Lomond, California: Genesis Press, 1972.

Lewis, Howard R., and Martha E. *The Medical Offenders.* New York: Simon & Schuster, 1970.

Liley, H.M.I., M.D., and Beth Day. *Modern Motherhood: Pregnancy, Childbirth and the Newborn Baby.* New York: Random House, 1969.

Llewellyn-Jones, Derek, M.D. *Everywoman and Her Body.* New York: Taplinger Publishing Company, 1971.

McCleary, Elliott H. *New Miracles of Childbirth.* New York: David McKay, 1974.

Meltzer, David. *Journal of the Birth.* Berkeley: Oyez Press, 1967.

Milinaire, Caterine. *birth.* New York: Harmony Books, 1974.

Montagu, Ashley. *The Natural Superiority of Women.* New York: The Macmillan Co., 1968.

Morris, Desmond. *The Naked Ape.* New York: McGraw-Hill Book Company, 1967.

Myles, Margaret F. *A Textbook for Midwives.* Edinburgh & London: Churchill Livingstone, 1972.

Newton, Niles, M.D. *Maternal Emotions.* New York: Paul E. Hoeber, Inc., 1955.

Reed, Constance, *Rapid Post Natal Figure Recovery.* Raritan, N.J.: Ortho Pharmaceutical Corporation, 1968.

Seaman, Barbara. *Free and Female.* New York: Coward, McCann & Geoghegan, Inc., 1972.

Shaw, Nancy Stoller, *Forced Labor: Maternity Care in the United States.* Elmsford, N.Y.: Pergamon Press, Inc. (Pergamon Studies in Critical Sociology), 1974.

Shideman, F.E., M.D., ed. *Take As Directed.* Minneapolis: Chemical Rubber Company, 1967.

Sweeney, William J., M.D., with Barbara Lang Stern. *Woman's Doctor.* New York: William Morrow, 1973.

Tanzer, Deborah, and Jean L. Block. *Why Natural Childbirth?* Garden City, New York: Doubleday & Co., 1972.

Thoms, Herbert, M.D. *Understanding Natural Childbirth.* New York: McGraw-Hill Book Co., Inc., 1950.

Vellay, Pierre, M.D. *Childbirth with Confidence.* New York: The Macmillan Co., 1969.

Weber, Laura E., M.D. *Between Us Women.* Garden City, New York: Doubleday & Co., Inc., 1962.

Wessel, Helen. *Natural Childbirth and the Family.* New York: Harper & Row, 1973.

White, Gregory J., M.D. *Emergency Childbirth.* Franklin Park, Ill.: Police Training Foundation, 1968.

Wigginton, Eliot. *Foxfire 2.* Garden City, New York: Anchor Press/Doubleday, 1973.

Wright, Erna. *The New Childbirth.* New York: Hart Publishing Co., 1966.

ARTICLES:

Abramson, Hilary. "Why can't mothers deliver their babies at home?" *The Sacramento Union,* May 5, 1974.

Arms, Suzanne. "How Hospitals Complicate Childbirth," *Ms.,* May, 1975.

Bradshaw, Susan Eisenhower. "Two Jam Jars, One Bucket, Two Pudding Basins" (Home Birth, a Personal Account), *The Saturday Evening Post,* May 1974.

Brazelton, T. Berry, M.D., "What Childbirth Drugs Can Do To Your Child," *Redbook,* February 1971.

Breu, G., ed., "Birth on the Kitchen Table," *Life,* Aug. 18, 1972.

Bridge, Peter. "1000 Midwife Dads Do It Themselves," *National Star,* November 9, 1974.

California Living. "What the Readers Think" (Childbirth) December 8, 1974.

Caruana, Stephanie. "Childbirth for the Joy of It," *Playgirl,* March 1974.

Comer, Nancy Axelrod. "Midwifery: Would You Let This Woman Deliver Your Child?" *Mademoiselle,* June 1973.

Connell, Elizabeth B., M.D. "The Modern Nurse-Midwife," *Redbook,* July 1974.

Coombs, Orde. "Some Babies Have to Be Born Twice," *Redbook,* October 1972.

Cromie, William J. "Drunken Roosters Aid in Motherhood Study," *The Sacramento Union,* January 16, 1974.

Dahlgren, Sune, M.D. "Reduction of Delivery Time by Cervical Dilatation Induced by Vibrations," *IRCS,* November 1973.

Di Cyan, Erwin. "Hospital Germs—Why They're Extra Deadly," *Family Weekly,* October 7, 1973.

Englund, Steven. " 'Birth Without Violence'," *The New York Times Magazine,* December 8, 1974.

Gittelson, Natalie. "Midwives?" *Harper's Bazaar,* June 1972.

Glamour. "What You Should Know About Having a Baby at Home," March 1974.

Good Housekeeping. "How Pregnancy Dangers Are Being Reduced," January 1974.

Gorbach, Arthur, M.D. "What to Expect During Labor and Delivery," *Redbook,* December 1972.

Hammer, Marian Behan. "The Midwife: A New Image," *Marriage,* December 1973.

Harmetz, Aljean. "The Way Childbirth *Really* Is," *Today's Health,* February 1972.

Harrison, Barbara Grizzuti. "Men Don't Know Nothin' 'Bout Birthin' Babies," *Esquire,* July 1973.

Jennings, C. Robert. "Eat Well With Adelle," *Cosmopolitan,* July 1972.

Klemesrud, Judy. "Why Women Are Losing Faith in Their Doctors," *McCall's,* June 1973.

Kramer, Linda. "Childbirth at Home," *The Sacramento Union,* October 27, 1974.

Landsberg, Michelle. "Your Gynecologist," *Chatelaine*, August 1973.

Lang, Dorothea M. "The Midwife Returns—Modern Style," *Parents*, October 1972.

Malloy, Michael T. "Prepared Childbirth: Sharing Love's Labor," *The National Observer*, August 30, 1971.

Maxwell AFB Hospital. "Information for Maternity Patients," Department of Obstetrics and Gynecology, Montgomery, Alabama, (N.D.)

McCann, Jean. "They Want to Have Their Babies at Home," *Marriage*, June 1971.

McLaughlin, Mary. "Now, an Alternative Obstetrical Style," *McCall's*, January 1973.

Meidus, Veronica. "Three Midwives Called Criminals: Attorney Cries 'Unconstitutional'," *The California Libertarian News*, July 4, 1974.

Milinaire, Caterine. "Home Birth: A Feast of Joy," *Vogue*, January 1, 1972.

National Foundation/March of Dimes. *Facts: 1975*.

Newsweek. "Sit Down, Have a Baby," May 21, 1973.

Newsweek. "Speedier, Easier Births with a Vibrator," July 30, 1973.

Newsweek. "Testing Baby's Brain," June 11, 1973.

Portland Times. "Infant's Father Unsure About Future Action," February 25, 1974.

Robinson, Donald. "The Newest Major Advances in Hospital Care," *Parade*, October 27, 1974.

Sacramento Bee. "Court Affirms Woman's Right to Pick Death," April 26, 1974.

Sacramento Bee. "Do Americans Starve? Yes, In Hospitals," March 29, 1974.

Sacramento Bee. "L A Women File Suit in Sterilization Case," November 21, 1974.

Sacramento Bee. "Tots Visit Maternity Ward," August 14, 1974.

Sacramento Union. "Malpractice Settlement May Top $1.2 Million," December 4, 1973.

Sander, Ellen. "Childbirth at Home," *Mademoiselle*, May 1972.

Schwabach, Deborah. "I Had My Baby in My Bedroom," *Redbook*, October 1968.

Shaw, Russell. "Controversy over Euthanasia," *The Catholic Free Press*, June 2, 1972.

Special Delivery. "New Demonstration Project Planned," Autumn 1974.

Stephen, Beverly. "Perinatal Care at Home," *San Francisco Chronicle*, October 4, 1973.

Streshinsky, Shirley. "Are You Safer With a Midwife?" *Ms.*, October 1973.

Sutherland, Donald. "Childbirth Is Not For Mothers Only," *Ms.*, May 1974.

Talbott, David, and Barbara Zheutlin, "The Legalities of Attending a Birth," *Rolling Stone*, May 23, 1974.

Time. "Return of the Midwife," November 20, 1972.

Torres, Tereska. "From Womb to World," *Ms.*, July 1974.

Tuck, Jay Nelson. "Make Room For Daddy," *Woman's Day*, (Medifacts), October 1972.

Von B., Marj. "Accused Santa Cruz Midwives Rally Defenders," *Watsonville (Calif.) Register-Pajaronian,* March 26, 1974.
Yost, Kaye. "At Home Or In The Hospital,"*California Living,* November 3, 1974.
Young, Patrick. "The Thoroughly Modern Midwife," *Saturday Review of Science,* September 2, 1972.

OTHER SOURCES:

Raymond Duff, M.D., Panel on Infant Euthanasia, *Tomorrow,* Tom Snyder, host. December 17, 1973.
Claude Edelman. *The First Days of Life* (film). Pierre Vellay, medical consultant. Suffolk, England: Boulton-Hawker Films.
Ashley Montagu. *The Tonight Show,* Johnny Carson, host. November 16, 1973. NBC Television Network.
Michael Whitt. Author interview with the physician in Point Reyes, California, May 10, 1974.
Santa Rosa, (Calif.) Public Health Department. Author interview with three midwives, December 11, 1973.
David Hartman. *Birth and Babies.* ABC Television Special, 1974.

INDEX